WITHDRAWN

Cystic Fibrosis

Papers by
Michael E. Fritz, Dorothy Martinez, A. D. Griffiths
et al.

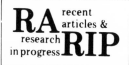

IN COOPERATION WITH THE
SMITHSONIAN SCIENCE INFORMATION EXCHANGE

Summaries of current research projects are included in the final section of this volume. Previously unpublished, these summaries were obtained from a search conducted by the Smithsonian Science Information Exchange, a national collection of information on ongoing and recently terminated research.

MSS Information Corporation
655 Madison Avenue, New York, N.Y. 10021

Library of Congress Cataloging in Publication Data
Main entry under title:

Cystic fibrosis.

   A collection of articles previously published
in various journals.
   1. Cystic fibrosis--Addresses, essays, lectures.
I. Fritz, Michael E [DNLM: 1. Cystic fibrosis--
Collected works. WI800 C999 1973]
RC857.C92   616.3'7   73-13832
ISBN 0-8422-7133-3

TABLE OF CONTENTS

CREDITS AND ACKNOWLEDGEMENTS

Biggar, W.D.; B. Holmes; and R.A. Good, "Opsonic Defect in Patients with Cystic Fibrosis of the Pancreas," *Proceedings of the National Academy of Sciences,* 1971, 68:1716-1719.

Cain, A.R.R.; A.M. Deall; and T.C. Noble, "Screening for Cystic Fibrosis by Testing Meconium for Albumin," *Archives of Disease in Childhood,* 1972, 47:131-132.

Cherry, James D.; Vernon J. Roden; Anthony J. Rejent; and Robert W. Dorner, "The Inhibition of Ciliary Activity in Tracheal Organ Cultures by Sera from Children with Cystic Fibrosis and Control Subjects," *The Journal of Pediatrics,* 1971, 79:937-942.

Cole, C.H.; and J.H. Dirks, "Changes in Erythrocyte Membrane ATPase in Patients with Cystic Fibrosis of the Pancreas," *Pediatric Research,* 1972, 6:616-621.

Davidson, A.G.F., "Diagnosis of Cystic Fibrosis," *British Medical Journal,* 1971, page 362.

Diaz, Federico; Luis L. Mosovich; and Erwin Neter, "Serogroups of *Pseudomonas aeruginosa* and the Immune Response of Patients with Cystic Fibrosis," *The Journal of Infectious Diseases,* 1970, 121:269-274.

Dolan, Thomas F., Jr.; and Lewis E. Gibson, "Complications of Iodide Therapy in Patients with Cystic Fibrosis," *The Journal of Pediatrics,* 1971, 79:684-687.

Featherby, Elizabeth A.; Tzong-Ruey Weng; and Henry Levison, "The Effect of Isoproterenol on Airway Obstruction in Cystic Fibrosis," *Canadian Medical Association Journal,* 1970, 102:835-841.

Fritz, Michael E.; Daniel B. Caplan; David Leever; and Jay Levitt, "Composition of Parotid Saliva on Different Days in Patients with Cystic Fibrosis," *American Journal of Diseases of Childhood,* 1972, 123: 116-117.

Graham, George G., "Buffered L-Arginine as Treatment for Cystic Fibrosis: State of the Evidence," *Pediatrics,* 1972, 49:471-472.

Greene, E.L.; S.P. Halbert; and J.C. Pallavicini, "Immunochemical Studies of Cystic Fibrosis Tissues: The Detection of Increased Concentrations of an Antigen Which Was Identified as C-Reactive Protein," *International Archives of Allergy and Applied Immunology,* 1971, 40: 184-196.

Griffiths, A.D.; and F.E. Bull, "Anomalous Sweat Chloride Levels in Cystic Fibrosis During Antibiotic Therapy," *Archives of Disease in Childhood,* 1972, 47:132-134.

Huang, Nancy N.; E. Joan Hiller; Carlos M. Macri; Marie Capitanio; and Kenneth R. Cundy, "Carbenicillin in Patients with Cystic Fibrosis: Clinical Pharmacology and Therapeutic Evaluation," *The Journal of Pediatrics*, 1971, 78:338-345.

Huang, Nancy N.; Carlos N. Macri; Joseph Girone; and Ann Sproul, "Survival of Patients with Cystic Fibrosis," *American Journal of Disease in Childhood*, 1970, 120:289-295.

Johnson, G. Frank; Max F. Thompson; S. Fetteroff; and A.N. Fasano, "Neutron Activation Analysis Technique for Nail Sodium Concentration in Cystic Fibrosis Patients," *Pediatrics*, 1971, 47:88-93.

Lifschitz, Martin I.; and Carolyn R. Denning, "Quantitative Interaction of Water and Cystic Fibrosis Sputum," *American Review of Respiratory Disease*, 1970, 102:456-458.

Martinez, Dorothy; and Anthony A. Silvidi, "A Nuclear Magnetic Resonance Study of Sodium in the Saliva of Patients with Cystic Fibrosis of the Pancreas," *Archives of Biochemistry and Biophysics*, 1972, 148: 224-227.

McCollum, Audrey T.; and Lewis E. Gibson, "Family Adaptation to the Child with Cystic Fibrosis," *The Journal of Pediatrics*, 1970, 77:571-578.

Motoyama, E.K.; L.E. Gibson; and C.J. Zigas, "Evaluation of Mist Tent Therapy in Cystic Fibrosis Using Maximum Expiratory Flow Volume Curve," *Pediatrics*, 1972, 50:299-306.

Šamánek, M.; J. Houštěk; V. Vávrová; C. Ruth; and O. Šnobl, "Distribution of Pulmonary Blood Flow in Children with Cystic Fibrosis," *Acta Pediatrica Scandinavica*, 1971, 60:149-157.

Schwartz, Robert H.; Douglas E. Johnstone; Douglas S. Holsclaw; and Richard R. Dooley, "Serum Precipitins to *Aspergillus fumigatus* in Cystic Fibrosis," *American Journal of Disease in Childhood*, 1970, 120:432-433.

Solomons, Clive C.; Ernest K. Cotton; Reuben Dubois; and Margo Pinney, "The Use of Buffered L-Arginine in the Treatment of Cystic Fibrosis," *Pediatrics*, 1971, 47:384-390.

Taylor, William F.; and Boulos Y. Qaqundah, "Neonatal Jaundice Associated with Cystic Fibrosis," *American Journal of Disease in Childhood*, 1972, 123:161-162.

Wilson, R.G., "Glycosaminoglycans in the Skin of Patients with Cystic Fibrosis of the Pancreas," *Clinica Chimica Acta*, 1972, 36:189-193.

Wright, Gordon L.T.; and James Harper, "Fusidic Acid and Lincomycin Therapy in Staphylococcal Infections in Cystic Fibrosis," *Lancet*, 1970, 1:9-11.

Zapletal, Alois; Etsuro K. Motoyama; Lewis E. Gibson; and Arend Bouhuys, "Pulmonary Mechanics in Asthma and Cystic Fibrosis," *Pediatrics*, 1971, 48:64-72.

PREFACE

Cystic Fibrosis (CF) is a autosomal recessive, metabolic disorder which presumably results from an unidentified enzyme defect. CF is characterized by both the retention of mucous secretions in the respiratory and digestive passages and an increased concentration of sodium and chloride in the sweat.

Although the basic inherited defect is apparently the same in all patients, the clinical manifestations vary a great deal, both in degree and timing. Symptoms of CF may present at birth or remain undetected until preschool age. The latter situation generally indicates a more favorable course for the disease.

A number of important nutritional symptoms observed in CF result from the obstruction of the pancreatic duct, depriving the child of pancreatic enzymes and bicarbonate. This in particular impedes the digestion of protein and fat. This impaired digestion usually leaves the child undernourished despite an increase in the total number of daily feedings. Retention of bronchial secretions tends to impede expiration and traps air in the chest, causing recurrent episodes of a choking cough. However, the diagnosis of CF should be suspected in any child not thriving on an adequate food intake, whether or not respiratory symptoms are present. The most consistent feature of the disease, and, therefore, one of the most useful in diagnosis, is the raised sodium and chloride content of sweat. Sodium concentration is generally three times that normally found.

Proper management of CF is often a complex procedure involving drugs, diet and strict supervision. CF greatly enhances the probability of respiratory infections, and the continuous administration of an antibiotic drug during the first few years of life is generally advisable. The nutritional symptoms associated with CF can often be controlled if replacement therapy with pancreatin is given with meals and diets are designed for maximum caloric intake. In addition, proper regulation of the environmental atmosphere by means of air purification and humidification has been shown to be of benefit to these patients.

Carriers of CF can usually be detected by use of ciliary inhibition tests, and proper genetic counseling of these individuals is of the utmost importance in preventing CF in offspring.

Life expectancy of patients with CF has been greatly improved by modern antibiotic treatment; however, this does not change the fact that cystic fibrosis is still fatal.

This collection of articles considers the chronic disorder cystic fibrosis from a diagnostic and therapeutic standpoint. Also included are articles emphasizing the complications of the disease as well as a number of general studies which should prove helpful in an overall understanding of the disease process.

Peter F. Weinheimer, Ph.D.
Ronald T. Acton, Ph.D.
September, 1973

General Studies

Composition of Parotid Saliva on Different Days in Patients With Cystic Fibrosis

Michael E. Fritz, DDS, PhD; Daniel B. Caplan, MD; David Leever; and Jay Levitt

Considerable interest[1] has often been generated by the apparent alteration of salivary electrolytes of patients with cystic fibrosis of the pancreas. Some workers[2-4] have claimed increases in flow rates of reflex or drug-stimulated parotid saliva in patients with cystic fibrosis; other workers[5,6] have not agreed. Similarly, utilizing various salivary stimuli, some authors have claimed increased electrolyte content in patients with cystic fibrosis while others[7] have disputed this claim. In all of these investigations, there has been no study of the saliva from the same individual collected on different days. The present investigation was conducted solely to determine to what extent the same patient, under the same experimental conditions, would exhibit similarity of response on two different days.

Methods

Subjects for this study were 11 children (six boys and five girls aged 6 to 15 years) with cystic fibrosis. Diagnostic criteria for cystic fibrosis were a clinical picture of respiratory disease and pancreatic insufficiency, and chloride concentration in sweat of greater than 80 mEq/liter. Collection of saliva was initially performed in each of these patients by direct cannulation of Stenson's duct on the right side of the patient by the technique of Mahan and Ramirez.[s] Following cannulation of Stenson's duct, saliva was collected under oil into tubes which exhibited tolerances of 0.1 ml at large volumes and tolerances of .01 ml at small volumes (0 to 1.0 ml). Collections were made in a quiet room, each child received careful instructions regarding the collection procedure, and frequent checks were made to ascertain that no saliva was leaking around the cannula. All collections were obtained between 10 AM and 3 PM, and each patient had been instructed not to eat any food from dinner the previous evening until collection time. Analyses were run on the day of collection and consisted of determinations of total osmolarity, sodium, potassium, chloride, and total protein.

Following cannulation of the salivary duct, unstimulated saliva was collected for a ten-minute interval commencing with the time the "dead space" of the tubing was filled. Following this, parotid fluid was stimulated by having each patient suck lemon flavored lozenges (Napoleons) which consist mainly of sugar and citric acid,[6] and saliva was again collected for ten minutes. Two to three months after the initial cannulation of Stenson's duct, each patient was appointed for a second cannulation. These patients had the same procedure done by the same investigators (D. L. and J. L.), utilizing the same experimental protocol in the same location. Analyses were done by the same techniques.

Results

Analyses of parotid saliva from the population of 11 subjects demonstrate the wide spread of values seen in saliva of patients with cystic fibrosis, and the data do not differ significantly from values for parotid saliva in other studies[3-7] dealing with patients with cystic fibrosis. The data obtained from eleven patients cannulated on two different occasions were subjected to analyses by paired differences and student t tests (Table). The data show no significant differences between populations with saliva obtained by lemon stimulation, but statistical differences in flow of saliva, sodium concentration, and

chloride concentration between nonstimulated salivas obtained on different collection days. The data also show that saliva collected during the second cannulation usually exhibited higher values for these factors.

Comment

The data obtained in the present study confirm the observation that sodium and chloride concentrations in saliva vary directly with flow rate. The data have also reconfirmed the large variance in individuals for flow rate of saliva and concentrations of various ions in saliva. The fact that values obtained in the present study do not differ significantly from those of reflex-stimulated parotid saliva obtained in other studies[3-7] with children with cystic fibrosis suggests similar populations are being analyzed.

In earlier studies the authors[4,5] have claimed a deficiency in ductal reabsorption of sodium in parotid saliva. This may be true only at high flow rates of saliva; in the present study a mean sodium concentration of unstimulated saliva obtained by direct cannulation was 4.35 mEq/liter, indicating that sodium in all probability is reabsorbed at slow salivary flow rates. Although collection of saliva in the present study was designed to be as close to basal conditions as possible, the fact that the patient knew the procedure would be undertaken and that there was a mechanical effect of the cannula would suggest that a true "resting" state was not achieved. The low value of sodium in these patients is, therefore, even more impressive, as these stimuli would have a tendency to increase flow rate and hence elevate the concentration of sodium.

Other than sodium and chloride concentrations in nonstimulated salivas, the remainder of the data collected from eleven pairs during both periods of nonstimulation and lemonstimulation fail to demonstrate any statistically significant differences.

Flow, Sodium, and Chloride Concentration of Saliva Collected on Two Different Days*

Patient	Nonstimulated 1			Nonstimulated 2			Lemon Stimulated 1			Lemon Stimulated 2		
	Flow (ml/min)	Sodium (mEq/Liter)	Chloride (mEq/Liter)	Flow (ml/min)	Sodium (mEq/Liter)	Chloride (mEq/Liter)	Flow (ml/min)	Sodium (mEq/Liter)	Chloride (mEq/Liter)	Flow (ml/min)	Sodium (mEq/Liter)	Chloride (mEq/Liter)
1	.025	5.6	16	.050	26.5	20	.26	9.0	22	.30	7.5	25
2	.030	6.5	22	.050	8.0	25	.70	11.5	31	1.20	24.0	39
3	.040	10.5	26	.050	9.5	28	.64	28.5	41	.60	15.5	37
4	.040	2.0	18	.050	5.0	19	.22	9.0	17	.45	31.0	29
5	.050	2.0	31	.055	7.5	30	.55	22.5	39	.40	17.5	34
6	.050	1.0	20	.065	8.0	22	.30	8.5	23	.41	26.5	29
7	.050	1.5	10	.050	1.6	14	.30	7.0	20	.37	9.0	26
8	.050	1.8	20	.040	2.5	21	.27	17.5	37	.35	19.0	39
9	.050	11.0	16	.140	37.5	19	.80	57.5	35	.45	44.0	34
10	.065	2.5	18	.090	3.5	21	.80	43.5	43	.65	57.0	40
11	.080	1.0	21	.080	6.0	19	.18	5.0	20	.30	20.5	24

* t_{flow} = 2.54 $P < 0.05$; t_{Na} = 2.39 $P < .05$; t_{Cl} = 3.14 $P < .05$; t_{flow} = 0.63 $P > 0.1$; t_{Na} = 1.27 $P > 0.1$; t_{Cl} = 1.58 $P > 0.1$.

These data however have an important bearing on the proper design of future experiments. The values for any individual fluctuate from day to day, whether saliva is collected under conditions of nonstimulation or reflex stimulation. Furthermore, the flow rate in response to reflex stimulation seems to be independent of the individual's basal value on that day (Table). In general, osmolarity and concentrations of sodium and chloride tended to follow the flow rate, whereas potassium was independent of flow rate. Concentration of protein also seems to be variable, failing to exhibit a correlation between basal value and increment after reflex stimulation on different days.

The findings in this report, therefore, cannot either reject or prove the hypothesis that there is a defect in the parotid gland duct system of children with cystic fibrosis. The data however do suggest that a reevaluation of experimental design should be considered.

This investigation was supported in part by Public Health Service grant 2879, grant 9835 from the National Cystic Fibrosis Research Foundation, and by student project funds of Emory University School of Dentistry.

References

1. diSant' Agnese PA, Grossman H, Darling RC, et al: Saliva, tears and duodenal contents in cystic fibrosis of the pancreas. Pediatrics 22:507-514, 1958.
2. Johnston WH: Salivary electrolytes in fibrocystic disease of the pancreas. Arch Dis Child 31:477-480, 1956.
3. Barbero GJ, Chernick W: Function of the salivary gland in cystic fibrosis of the pancreas. Pediatrics 22:945-952, 1958.
4. Marmar J, Barbero GJ, Sabinga MS: The pattern of parotid gland secretion in cystic fibrosis of the pancreas. Gastroenterology 50:551-556, 1966.
5. Chauncey HH, Levine DM, Kass G, et al: Parotid gland secretory rate and electrolyte concentration in children with cystic fibrosis. Arch Oral Biol 7:707-713, 1962.
6. Kutscher AH, Mandel ID, Thompson RH, et al: Parotid saliva in cystic fibrosis: I. Flow rate. Amer J Dis Child 110:643-645, 1965.
7. Mandel ID, Thompson RH, Wotman S, et al: Parotid saliva in cystic fibrosis: II. Electrolytes and protein-bound carbohydrates. Amer J Dis Child 110:646-651, 1965.
8. Mahan PE, Ramirez GA: Reliable method of collecting parotid saliva from human subjects. J Dent Res 43:1256, 1964.

A Nuclear Magnetic Resonance Study of Sodium in the Saliva of Patients with Cystic Fibrosis of the Pancreas

DOROTHY MARTINEZ AND ANTHONY A. SILVIDI

Cystic fibrosis is a hereditary disease which is characterized by a generalized dysfunction of the exocrine glands. The basic molecular defect of this disease has not yet been determined (1). Clinical effects of the disease encompass chronic pulmonary disease, pancreatic deficiency, salivary gland involvement, and sweat gland abnormality (2). One manifestation of this disease is an increase of sodium and chloride in the sweat and mixed saliva of CFP patients (3, 4). In this investigation, we are particularly concerned with Na increase in the saliva. The increase in Na concentration is thought to be due not to the initial concentration of Na secreted, but to the fact that in a normal individual much of the Na initially secreted is reabsorbed in the duct of the gland before final secretion of the

14

fluid (sweat or saliva). Apparently there is something which prevents this reabsorption of Na in the CFP patient (3). Determination of the molecular defect preventing reabsorption of Na would aid in an eventual understanding of the basic defect of this disease. Spock (5) has reported that the defect preventing reabsorption of Na may result from an alteration of cell membrane permeability. Mangos, McSherry, and Benke (3, 6) have reported finding a "factor" in the saliva of CFP patients that causes inhibition of Na transport. They (3, 6) also indicate that inhibition of sodium reabsorption occurs by an action other than inhibition of the activity of ATPase, an enzyme known to be involved in Na transport across biological membranes.

The purpose of this investigation was to determine whether the saliva of CFP patients contained some factor which was complexing the Na and thus preventing the Na from acting as a free ion with respect to its permeability to the salivary duct membrane. Na binding (or complexing) appeared to be a definite possibility considering the greatly decreased transport of Na across the duct membrane as manifested by the significantly greater Na concentration in saliva of CFP patients compared to controls, and also in consideration of the possible complex formation between sodium and the abnormal proteins and carbohydrates (7, 8) found in saliva of CFP patients. Nuclear Magnetic Resonance (nmr) is an experimental tool uniquely suited to this purpose. In a sample containing both Na in a complexed state (bound to some large molecule), and Na existing as a free ion, the nmr will detect only the free ionic Na (9) if the free Na is exchanging, into an environment in which the line is very broad, at a rate which is slow compared to the line width. If the exchange rate were rapid, the bound Na could contribute to the observed resonance by broadening the line or by shifting its position. Thus, we have a method for determining if the Na in the saliva of CFP patients is prevented from reabsorption because it is bound to a large molecule and, therefore, cannot move freely

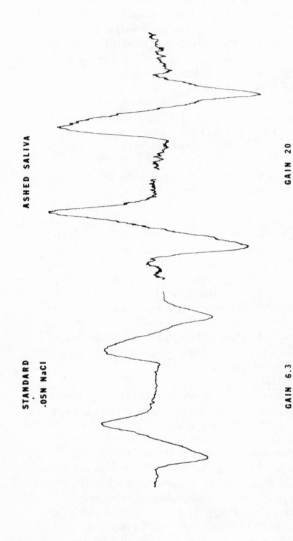

STANDARD
.05N NaCl

ASHED SALIVA

GAIN 6.3

GAIN 20

FIG. 1. Representative nmr traces of the Standard sodium chloride solution and saliva. The line widths as determined from the derivative curves of the intact and ashed saliva of both normal controls and CFP patients was 0.1 G. No detectable change in chemical shift was noted in any of these traces.

16

across the duct membrane. If the Na in the saliva of CFP patients is found to be completely ionic or no different in binding from control subjects, then the defect inhibiting Na transport must lie elsewhere.

MATERIALS AND METHODS

A Varian (Varian Associates, Palo Alto, Calif.) model No. VF-16C wide-line spectrometer set to give the derivative of the resonance curve with a magnetic field strength of approximately 7000 G, and a radio frequency of approximately 7880 kHz was used to obtain all experimental data. The 4–8 MHz probe was used throughout.

Fresh whole mixed saliva samples of approximately 2 cm^3 were obtained, by expectoration, from controls (normal, healthy subjects—both male and female of various ages), and from patients diagnosed as having CFP. These samples were centrifuged at 500g for 5 min and the supernatant fluid was transferred to Vycor tubes of 1.5 cm diameter. Two traces of the nmr spectra of each sample were recorded and the peak-to-peak height of the derivative curves were averaged in order to reduce instrumental noise. Some of the fresh saliva samples were then heated in the same Vycor test tubes to 100° for approximately 1 hr. After the samples were cooled, additional nmr spectra were obtained. Some of the samples were reheated to dryness at approximately 100°, and then ashed at 300° (still in the same Vycor tubes). The ashed samples were then redissolved in HCl. Care was taken to assure that the volume of the ashed sample in HCl was the same as the volume of the fresh saliva sample before ashing. NMR spectra were obtained for these ashed samples. NMR spectra of a standard solution of 0.05 N NaCl were recorded before and after each set of saliva samples. The nmr apparatus was retuned after inserting each saliva and each standard sample. Representative nmr traces from our measurements of saliva are shown in Fig. 1. Calculations of free Na were based on the experimental evidence (9, 10) that the peak-to-peak height of the derivative curve is directly proportional to the concentration of free Na in the sample. It has also been demonstrated that when Na is complexed with an ion exchange resin, the nmr spectrum of Na is broadened so greatly that it becomes invisible (11). We are, therefore, assuming that the only Na in the saliva which gives rise to a resonance curve is the Na in free solution. Such an assumption has been made in other nmr studies (9, 10, 12, 13) of Na complexing in living cells and body fluids. In order to

TABLE I

Na Concentrations in Milliequivalents Liter for Fresh and Ashed Saliva from CFP Patients and Controls. Values in Parentheses are Probabilities Determined from t Distribution

		Fresh saliva	Ashed saliva	(Ashed—Fresh)
A. CFP patients		28.8	29.7	+0.9
		12.3	11.9	−0.4
		12.7	12.4	−0.3
		37.5	41.5	+4.0
		12.4	14.2	+1.8
		19.1	22.4	+3.3
	Avg	20.5		+1.6 (>0.95)
B. Controls		2.8	3.7	+0.9
		5.1	5.4	+0.3
		7.1	7.2	+0.1
		7.5	8.7	+1.2
		8.5	9.9	+1.4
		6.9	7.1	+0.2
	Avg	6.3		+0.7 (>0.995)

further check the accuracy of determining total Na concentrations by the ashing methods described here, we used a flame photometer and also a wet ashing (with concd. H_2SO_4) procedure followed by nmr analysis to determine total Na concentration. All three methods yielded comparable results.

RESULTS AND DISCUSSION

Table I gives the Na concentration in milliequivalents/liter of fresh saliva and ashed saliva for both CFP patients and controls. The Na concentration of the ashed sample is the total sodium in the sample (both free and bound). As expected, the average Na concentration in fresh saliva for CFP patients of 20.5 meq/liter is significantly greater than the average value for the controls of 6.3 meq/l. We also see that the average increase in Na from fresh to ashed saliva for CFP patients is 1.6 meq/liter or 7.6%. For controls, the average increase is 0.7 meq/liter or 10.9%. After taking into account the reproducibility of nmr traces, the error in determining Na concentration by this method and possible losses in ashing procedures, we find that the maximum possible

TABLE II

Na CONCENTRATIONS IN MILLIEQUIVALENTS LITER FOR FRESH SALIVA AND SALIVA HEATED TO 100° FROM CFP PATIENTS AND CONTROLS. VALUES IN PARENTHESES ARE PROBABILITIES DETERMINED FROM t DISTRIBUTION

	Fresh saliva	Heated to 100°	(Heated—Fresh)
A. CFP patients	14.1	17.9	+3.8
	21.3	24.0	+2.7
	9.3	9.6	+0.4
	28.4	30.3	+1.9
	13.1	16.4	+3.3
	20.9	24.8	+3.9
	13.0	16.3	+3.3
	15.0	16.5	+1.5
	28.8	31.6	+2.8
	12.3	12.9	+0.6
	12.7	12.2	−0.5
	37.5	34.0	−3.5
	12.4	12.7	+0.3
	19.1	20.6	+1.5
	Avg 18.4		+1.6 (>0.995)
B. Controls	8.0	6.6	−1.4
	8.2	8.0	−0.2
	3.5	4.0	+0.5
	5.3	4.6	−0.7
	2.8	2.8	0.0
	5.1	5.3	+0.2
	7.1	6.8	−0.3
	7.5	8.1	+0.6
	8.5	8.5	0.0
	6.9	6.2	−0.7
	Avg 6.3		−0.2 (>0.95)

experimental error is approximately 12%. Both values (7.6% and 10.9%) are within this experimental error. We, therefore, conclude that, within experimental error, there is no difference in Na binding in the saliva of CFP patients compared to controls.

Mangos, McSherry, and Benke (3) have reported that the "factor" which was preventing sodium reabsorption was destroyed by heating the saliva to 100°. We, therefore, checked to see if there was a difference in Na binding in saliva of CFP patients that would be evident after heating the saliva to 100°. The results of this investigation are shown in Table II. We again see, as expected, that the average value of Na concentration of 18.4 meq/liter was significantly greater in the saliva of the CFP as compared to a control average value of 6.3 meq/liter. Upon heating the saliva to 100°, we find an average increase of 1.6 meq/liter or 8.5% for CFP patients, and an average decrease of 0.2 meq/liter or 3.0% for controls. Both of these values are within experimental errors. We therefore, conclude that Na binding cannot account for the loss of inhibition of Na transport reported by Mangos, McSherry, and Benke (3) when saliva samples were heated to 100°.

The results of these investigations suggest that there is no difference in the binding of Na in the saliva of CFP patients as compared to controls. In both cases most of the Na is not exchanging slowly onto a macromolecule. Similar conclusions regarding the diffusibility of sodium in isolated submaxillary secretions of patients with cystic fibrosis and normal controls have been reached by Potter and co-workers (14). Therefore, the Na transport mechanism of inhibition in the saliva of patients with CFP cannot be related to binding of the Na and thus inhibiting reabsorption in the duct of the gland. These conclusions are consistent with the speculation of Mangos and McSherry (6) that the Na transport inhibitory factor may be a strongly basic macromolecule that interacts with the cell membrane of transporting epithelia and causes a defect in the reabsorption of Na. The results here are also consistent with Spock's view (5) that a humoral substance within the cell results in increased metabolic activity within the cell with subsequent alteration of cell membrane permeability. Both of these views (5, 6) support a change in the membrane. By eliminating the possibility of a change in Na reabsorption due to Na binding, our results also lend support to this view.

ACKNOWLEDGMENT

We wish to thank Dr. J. Potter of Children's Hospital, Akron, Ohio, for aid in obtaining samples of saliva from patients with CFP.

REFERENCES

1. TALAMO, R. C., *Calif. Med.* **110**, 432–434 (1969).
2. DiSANT'AGNESE, P. A., Research on Pathogenesis of Cystic Fibrosis (1964).
3. MANGOS, J. A., McSHERRY, N. R., AND BENKE, P. J., *Pediat. Res.* **1**, 436–442 (1967).
4. MANGOS, J. A., AND McSHERRY, N. A., *Science* **158**, 135–136 (1967).
5. SPOCK, A., *Minn. Med.* **52**, 1429–1432 (1969).
6. MANGOS, J. A., AND McSHERRY, N. R., *Pediat. Res.* **2**, 378–384 (1968).
7. CHERNICK, W. S., AND BARBERO, G. J., *Ann. N.Y. Acad. Sci.* **106**, 698–798 (1963).
8. ZIPKIN, I. HAWKINS, G. R. DAMERGIS, J. A. GUGLER, E., SWERDLOW, H., DiSANT, AGNESE, P. Cystic Fibrosis Club Abstr., 11th Annu. Meet., p. 57 (1970).
9. MARTINEZ, D., SILVIDI, A. A., STOKES, R. M., *Biophys. J.* **9**, No. 10, 1256–1260 (1969).
10. COPE, F. W., *Proc. Nat. Acad. Sci. U.S.A.* **54**, 225 (1965).
11. JARDETSKY, O., AND WERTZ, J. E., *J. Amer. Chem. Soc.* **82**, 318 (1960).
12. ROTUNNO, C. A., AND KOWALEWSKI, V., AND CECEYIDO, N., *Biochem. Biophys. Acta* **135**, 170 (1967).
13. JARDETSKY, O., AND WERTZ, J. E., *Amer. J. Physiol.* **187**, 608 (1956).
14. POTTER, J. L., personal communication.

Anomalous Sweat Chloride Levels in Cystic Fibrosis During Antibiotic Therapy

A. D. GRIFFITHS and F. E. BULL

It is becoming increasingly common to confirm the diagnosis of cystic fibrosis by using a skin chloride electrode, and estimation of the sodium content of sweat is now often omitted.

The following case report concerns a child with proven cystic fibrosis in whom raised sweat sodium but normal sweat chloride levels were obtained while she was receiving cloxacillin.

Possible explanations for the findings are discussed and attention is drawn to their implications in relation to screening programmes for cystic fibrosis.

Method

Sweat was collected on to sodium chloride free Whatman No. 40 filter paper squares (3·5 cm) after conventional pilocarpine iontophoresis using the EMI sweat unit.* The sweat was eluted with 2·0 ml deionized water. 100 mg of sweat was accepted as the minimum weight for analysis as suggested by Varley (1967). Sodium was estimated by flame photometry and chloride by a modified Schales and Schales technique.

The mean and normal range for sweat electrolytes at this hospital are as follows: *sodium*: mean 21·1 mEq/l., range 5–45 mEq/l. (n = 56); *chloride*: mean 13·6 mEq/l., range 2–40 mEq/l. (n = 55).

---

*EMI—Electromedical Supplies (Greenham) Ltd.

Case Report

The infant was delivered by caesarian section after a pregnancy complicated by pre-eclamptic toxaemia, birthweight 2·3 kg. She was the youngest of three sibs, one of whom has diabetes mellitus. On two occasions in the early months of life she was admitted to an isolation hospital with suspected gastroenteritis, and at the age of 10 months presented with a history of recurrent respiratory infections and persistent stridor. Her chest x-ray was normal and a diagnosis of congenital laryngeal stridor was made. The stridor gradually subsided over the next 14 months.

She was referred again at the age of 3 years with rectal prolapse and a history of passing loose, bulky, grey stools. Coeliac disease was suspected and she was admitted for observation. There was no pot belly or muscle wasting and she was discharged after a few days as her stools were thought to be normal. A total faecal fat excretion of 43·2 g over a 5-day period was recorded at this time, but no further action was taken. The rectal prolapse remained troublesome for the next 12 months.

She was next referred at the age of 9 years to the chest clinic with a 3-month history of cough. A chest x-ray then showed increased lung markings and fibrosis in the right upper zone. Breathing exercises were started and antibiotics advised during the winter months. She did not improve over the next 2 years and was admitted to the regional chest hospital in July 1970, at the age of 11 years, with suspected bronchiectasis. When she was first seen by one of us (A.D.G.) in October 1970, she was febrile (temperature 38 °C), dyspnoeic, slightly jaundiced, and many spider naevi were visible. The sputum was frankly purulent, her fingers clubbed, there was moderate intercostal insuction, and crepitations were audible over the whole chest. The abdomen was distended and both liver and spleen were palpably enlarged. A clinical diagnosis of cystic fibrosis was made and sweat tests arranged. The quantities of sweat obtained initially were low. On 29 October 1970 she was transferred to this hospital for further investigation. The results were as follows: Hb 11·6 g, ESR 76 mm, WBC 6900/mm³ (73% polymorphs), sputum cultured a coagulase positive staphylococcus and *H. influenzae*. Bone age normal. Faecal fat excretion over 3 days 8·6 g as stearic acid/24 hours. Plasma proteins 7·3 g/100 ml, albumin 5·5 g/100 ml, IgG 2200 mg/100 ml, IgA >500 mg/100 ml, IgM 190 mg/100 ml. Total bilirubin 1·0 mg/100 ml, SGOT 112 RF units/ml, SGPT 44RF units/ml, LDH 420 BB untis/ml. The results of several sweat tests are shown in the Table. She was treated with various antibiotics (see Table), inhalations, and physiotherapy, and discharged 1 month later, by which time she had improved though crepitations persisted at the left base.

She was readmitted on 2 further occasions with exacerbations of her chest infection and during the latter suffered a massive haemoptysis and died 13 February 1971, at the age of 11 years 8 months.

23

TABLE
Sweat Electrolytes

Date	Weight of Sweat (mg)	Sodium (mEq/l.)	Chloride (mEq/l.)	Method	Place	Antibiotic Therapy
21.10.70	26	29	19	Iontophoresis	Nevill Hall Hospital	Nil (cloxacillin discontinued 8.10.70)
28.10.70	66	106	12	Iontophoresis	Nevill Hall Hospital	Cloxacillin 125 mg 6-hourly (begun 24.10.70)
30.10.70	258	103	5	Iontophoresis	Nevill Hall Hospital	Cloxacillin 500 mg 6-hourly
4.11.70	77	113	8	Iontophoresis	Nevill Hall Hospital	
11.11.70	108	99	6	Iontophoresis	Nevill Hall Hospital	Cloxacillin 500 mg 6-hourly + Ampicillin 500 mg 6-hourly
17.11.70	—	—	14·5	Skin chloride electrode	East Glamorgan Hospital	
25.11.70	70	{107 102	150 Insufficient	Iontophoresis	Nevill Hall Hospital	Nil (previous antibiotic stopped 24.11.70)
26.11.70	—	—	{90 84 72	Iontophoresis Skin chloride electrode	East Glamorgan Hospital Llandough Hospital	No antibiotics
5.12.70	159	85	75	Iontophoresis	Nevill Hall Hospital	Carbenicillin 500 mg 6-hourly (begun 27.11.70)

24

Necropsy revealed saccular bronchiectasis of the right upper lobe, haemorrhagic consolidation of both lower lobes, and purulent secretion in the bronchi. There was moderate ascites, and the liver, which weighed 1360 g, was grossly nodular and tawny green in colour. The pancreas was of fibrous fatty structure with small cysts containing thick mucinous secretions. Histologically the pancreas showed the typical features of cystic fibrosis and sections of the liver revealed fibrosis of the portal tracts, the bile ducts being dilated with dark bile.

Discussion

Altogether 9 sweat tests were performed on this child and the results are summarized in the Table. The weight of sweat obtained in the initial test, on 21 October 1970, was small and the results therefore questionable, but in the following 5 tests a markedly raised sodium concentration in the presence of a normal chloride level was consistently demonstrated.

Apparent disproportionate rise of the sodium content of sweat might occur if the sample is contaminated with sodium containing dusting powders which have been applied to the skin. This possibility can be excluded in the present case as care was taken to cleanse the skin thoroughly before the test, and in any event it would fail to explain the concurrent low chloride levels unless it was assumed either that the child did not have cystic fibrosis, or that she had, but without sweat gland involvement. Both these assumptions are invalid, as the diagnosis of cystic fibrosis was confirmed at necropsy and involvement of the sweat glands shown by subsequent sweat tests at this and other hospitals.

The possibility of a temporary laboratory error in chloride assessment has to be considered, but it is unlikely as the low level was also confirmed at another hospital using a skin chloride electrode.

All the low sweat chloride levels were recorded during a period when the child was receiving cloxacillin sodium, and when this drug was discontinued the discrepancy between sodium and chloride levels disappeared. It was not possible to see whether reintroduction of cloxacillin would reproduce the sweat anomaly in the present case as the organisms in the sputum had become resistant to this antibiotic, and death occurred shortly afterwards.

Although the sweat abnormality might be due to as yet unknown factors, the temporal association with cloxacillin administration suggests a causative relation, and it is tempting to speculate that the anomaly was produced by the substitution of the cloxacillin radicle for the chloride ion in the sweat during the period of therapy.

While it is possible that these findings are peculiar to this case, until further study has been undertaken it is suggested that the results of sweat tests in children with suspected cystic fibrosis be reviewed in the light of any antibiotic therapy which they may be receiving; this applies especially where a sweat chloride only is assessed, as in screening programmes utilizing a skin chloride electrode.

The authors thank Dr. P. Bray and Mr. R. Christopher-Prosser for arranging sweat tests at Llandough and East Glamorgan Hospitals.

REFERENCE

Varley, H. (1967). *Practical Clinical Biochemistry*, 4th ed., p. 426. Heinemann, London and New York.

GLYCOSAMINOGLYCANS IN THE SKIN OF PATIENTS WITH CYSTIC FIBROSIS OF THE PANCREAS

INTRODUCTION

In 1968 Johansen et al.[1] postulated that the basic defect in the disease cystic fibrosis of the pancreas (CF) expressed itself as an inhibition of fluid movement from the extracellular space across secretory epithelia throughout the body. They further suggested that the defect may be related to an abnormality in extracellular muco-substances, possibly in the abnormal distribution of chemically normal glycosamino-glycans (GAG's) or in a chemical abnormality in one of the GAG constituents. This might lead to changes in the three-dimensional network of these complex, negatively-charged macromolecules with consequent effects on the "porosity" of the region to the movement of small ions and water.

This paper describes investigations on the GAG composition of skin from some children suffering from CF, and of skin from normal children. Skin was chosen because it is the most readily obtainable tissue containing exocrine glands, and there is a distinctive disturbance in the normal production of sweat electrolytes in CF.

EXPERIMENTAL

Material

Skin was obtained for biopsy from 30 children with CF, who were attending the outpatient department at the Royal Children's Hospital in Melbourne, from 20

27

children who were not suffering from any illness and from 8 children with chronic illnesses. The procedure, and reasons for it were explained to the parents, and also, where possible, to the children. Only willing volunteers were sampled. All procedures were carried out by the medical staff of the Gastroenterological Research Unit.

Specimens were taken from the flexor surface of the forearm under local anaesthesia (1% Xylocaine), and were either processed immediately, or wrapped in Parafilm (to prevent water loss) and stored at -20 °C. Average wet weight of these specimens was 5 mg.

Methods

The specimen was cut into small pieces, one piece of which was assayed for hydroxyproline content by a minor modification of the method of Grunbaum and Glick[2]. The remainder was extracted with chloroform–methanol (2:1, v/v), to remove lipids, and then dehydrated in a vacuum dessicator over phosphorous pentoxide. The general techniques employed for the extraction of GAG's from the fat-free dry skin were those used by Thunell[3] for blood vessel walls*. One to three milligrams of dried defatted skin were incubated with 1 ml EDTA/cysteine (0.05 M EDTA, plus 0.0025 M cysteine hydrochloride in water, adjusted to pH 7.3 with sodium hydroxide). Papain suspension were added (10 μl of a solution containing 13 mg/ml), and the mixture incubated for 8 h at 37°.

GAG's were precipitated by adding 5 ml of 1% cetylpyridinium chloride (CPC) in 0.02 M sodium chloride, allowing the GAG's-CPC complex to form overnight at 30°. The complex was recovered by centrifuging at approximately 1500 g for 15 min at room temperature.

After careful decantation of the supernatant, the precipitate was dissolved in 40 μl isopropanol and 200 μl 60% v/v isopropanol–water was used to wash down the walls of the tube. Any turbidity of the solution was cleared by the addition of either isopropanol or water.

The sodium salts of the GAG's were precipitated with 2 ml ethanol and 50 μl 25% w/v aqueous sodium acetate. The tubes were stood overnight at 4–6° and the NaGAGs recovered by centrifugation as before. Following decantation and draining the final precipitate was taken up in 500 μl water and stored frozen until required.

The GAG content of this solution was estimated by assaying for uronic acid by the method of Brown[4], and hexosamine by the method described by Antonopoulos *et al.*[5], after acid hydrolysis and ion exchange chromatography as described by Boas[6].

Results

It was not possible to carry out all assays on some of the smaller specimens. The age distribution of the CF group was 8.3 years $\pm$ 4.2 (standard deviation) and that of the normal group was 8.9 years $\pm$ 3.1.

There was considerable overlap of values in both these groups for all parameters tested and only the differences in mean values were studied statistically (Table I). The statistical methods employed take into account the small number of specimens and the possibility of differences in variances[7].

---

* The modifications to analytical methods and the experiments carried out to modify Thunell's technique for use in this situation are fully covered in a thesis submitted by the author to the University of Melbourne as partial requirement for the degree of Master of Science.

TABLE I

	Normal			CF			
Skin:							
dried defatted weight*	33.6	± 1.6	(17)**	47.2	± 3.4	(21)	P<0.001***
hydroxyproline content+	52.9	± 2.9	(20)	44.5	± 2.9	(21)	P>0.05
GAGs:							
uronic acid content+	1.98	± 0.11	(20)	2.88	± 0.24	(28)	P<0.005
uronic acid content†	0.039	± 0.002	(20)	0.060	± 0.006	(19)	P<0.005
hexosamine content+	2.17	± 0.26	(17)	2.21	± 0.22	(16)	P>0.05
hexosamine content†	0.041	± 0.004	(17)	0.057	± 0.008	(13)	P>0.05

Statistical analysis of the results was carried out as described by Bailey.[7]

    * as a percentage of the wet weight
    ** mean ± standard error of the mean (number of specimens assayed)
    *** P is the probability of the difference between the mean values occurring by chance.
    + μg/mg dried, defatted wight
    † μg/μg hydroxyproline

    The difference in dried defatted weight of the skin specimens of the two groups was difficult to interpret as an aqueous anaesthetic had been injected just before the skin had been taken for biopsy.

    Hydroxyproline content was used as the basis of comparison of the parameters because
(a) it represents more truly the fibrous element (collagen) of the connective tissue being examined,
(b) the mean values between the two groups were not significantly different and,
(c) analysis of the variation of hydroxyproline with age showed that the regression lines for both groups are not significantly different either from zero or from each other, at the 5% level.

    This parameter may well fill the criteria of Langgård et al.[8] that "when tissue-analytical data are to be presented, a substance which is unaffected during the experimental conditions should be searched for".

    A statistically significant increase in the mean uronic acid value of the CF group compared with the normal group was noted whether this parameter was related to dried defatted weight or to hydroxyproline content. On the other hand no difference was noted in mean hexosamine content of the two groups.

    The choice of normal children for the control group in this study may not be valid as any changes in connective tissue GAG's may only be due to non-specific changes associated with chronic illness in general, rather than to cystic fibrosis of the pancreas specifically. An attempt was made to collect skin specimens from a group of children suffering from chronic illnesses other than CF, and whose height and weight were of the same order. Only a small group were available for study as many children with illnesses such as chronic renal failure and chronic hepatic cirrhosis do not survive to the same ages as CF patients. The mean age of a small group of 8 patients was 6 years, with a range of 6 months to 11 years. Hexosamine estimations were not performed on the extracted GAG's in this group. Statistically the results shown in Table II suffer because of the small numbers, but I think that the chronically ill group of children are more likely to be part of the normal population than to be part of the CF population. This suggests that the differences shown in Table I are associated with CF.

TABLE II

	Chronically ill group		Comparison with	
			CF group	Normal group
Skin:				
dried, defatted weight*	28.6 ± 1.3	(8)**	$P < 0.001$***	$P < 0.1 > 0.05$
hydroxyproline content+	56.9 ± 2.9	(7)	$P < 0.05 > 0.025$	$P < 0.5 > 0.4$
GAGs:				
uronic acid content+	3.01 ± 0.49	(8)	$P > 0.8$	$P < 0.1 > 0.05$
uronic acid content†	0.056 ± 0.022	(7)	$P > 0.6$	$P < 0.2 > 0.1$

For details see Table I.

Analysis of the variation of uronic acid content of the skin in the CF, and normal groups, with age show regressions which are neither significantly different from zero nor from each other (at the 5% level).

No attempt was made to assess the severity of their disease in the CF group, at the time of sampling. All children had been diagnosed clinically and had elevated sweat electrolytes. Treatment at the time included pancreatic supplements, antibiotics, aerosol inhalations and salt supplements.

DISCUSSION

In skin, uronic acid has been found only in the glycosaminoglycans of the connective tissue. An increase in skin uronic acid level in the CF group indicates an increase in GAG's. On the other hand hexosamines, the other major components of GAG's, are found in other molecules in skin tissue, e.g. glycoproteins, and the increase in hexosamine content equivalent to that of the uronic acids may be masked by alterations in other components.

The results reported here are at variance with those of Langgård et al.[9], who found a decrease in uronic acid and hexosamine content of skin from children with CF compared with normal skin. However their material was obtained from the thigh under general anaesthesia, and GAG's were not extracted from the skin, the components being assayed after acid hydrolysis. Only five children with CF were studied by these authors but they did look at the electrolyte composition of the skin and suggested a correlation between this and the changes in uronic acid and hexosamine content.

The two major GAG's of skin are dermatan sulphate and hyaluronic acid, although there have been reports of other GAG's in minor quantities[10]. Attempts were made to see whether either of these major components was responsible for the increase in uronic acid.

Separations were attempted by ion exchange, fractionation according to critical salt concentration, electrophoresis on cellulose acetate and paper, and thin layer chromatography. Results were not reproducible although Gardell and his co-workers have claimed to separate the GAG's in histological sections of nasal cartilage[5]. It was not found possible, using their techniques, to show any differences in the GAG composition of the skin in the CF and normal groups.

Increased skin GAG content may result from an increased rate of production compared with degradation, or a decreased rate of degradation. If the former were the case, increased urinary excretion of the degradation products of GAG's might be expected. Urinary excretion of GAG's was studied in a group of 10 CF children, 11 normals and 12 children with one of the mucopolysaccharidoses.* All the children in the latter group excreted considerable amounts of GAG-like material as would be expected from patients with a disease characterised by considerable tissue accumulation of GAG due to faulty degradation of tissue GAG's[11]. The CF group did not excrete any more GAG-like material than the normal group. However, the methods of extraction and assay of urine material may not have been sensitive enough to detect small changes.

Recently hypotheses for the cause of some of the "storage diseases" have been put forward, implicating defective degradation of GAG's by tissue lysosomal enzymes. Deficiencies of α-mannosidase[12] and α-fucosidase[13] have been described in two rare variants of the mucopolysaccharide syndrome and a β-galactosidase deficiency has been reported in Hurler's syndrome[14]. A study of skin lysosomal acid hydrolases has been undertaken to see if alteration in activity of some of the lysosomal acid hydrolases may account for the observed increase in uronic acid containing material in CF skin[15].

The increase in skin uronic acid content reported here must be viewed with the mass of other biochemical abnormalities already documented in CF[1]. It seems likely that these changes are secondary to the unknown basic defect but may be responsible for some of the abnormalities in water and electrolyte movements as suggested by Johansen[1].

REFERENCES

1 P. G. JOHANSEN, C. M. ANDERSON AND B. HADORN, Lancet, i (1968) 455.
2 B. W. GRUNBAUM AND D. GLICK, Arch. Biochem. Biophys., 65 (1956) 260.
3 S. THUNELL, Acta Univ. Lund., 2 (1967) 1.
4 A. H. BROWN, Arch. Biochem. Biophys., 11 (1946) 269.
5 C. A. ANTONOPOULOS, S. GARDELL, J. A. SZIRMAI AND E. R. DE TYSSONSK, Biochim. Biophys. Acta, 83 (1963) 1.
6 N. F. BOAS, J. Biol. Chem., 204 (1953) 553.
7 N. T. J. BAILEY, Statistical Methods in Biology, English University Press, London, 1959.
8 H. LANGGÅRD AND E. SECHER-HANSEN, Acta Pharmacol. Toxicol., 25 (1967) 267.
9 H. LANGGÅRD, H. HAASE AND E. W. FLENSBORG, Acta Paediat. Scand., 57 (1968) 255.
10 R. M. PEARCE, in R. W. JEANLOZ AND E. A. BALAZ (Eds.), The Amino Sugars, Vol. 2A, Academic Press, New York 1965, p. 149.
11 H. MUIR, Amer. J. Med., 47 (1969) 673.
12 P. A. ÖCKERMAN, Lancet, ii (1967) 239.
13 P. DURRAND, C. BORRONE AND G. DELLA CELLA, J. Pediat., 75 (1969) 665.
14 M. McBRINN, S. OKADA, M. WOOLLACOTT, V. PATEL, M. W. HO, A. L. TAPPEL AND J. S. O'-BRIEN, New Eng. J. Med., 281 (1969) 338.
15 R. G. WILSON, Clin. Chim. Acta, 36 (1972) 113.

---

* This, and the work on the attempted fractionation of skin GAG's, is fully reported in the thesis previously mentioned.

Changes in Erythrocyte Membrane ATPase in Patients with Cystic Fibrosis of the Pancreas

C. H. Cole and J. H. Dirks

Introduction

Patients with CFP have a defect in net sodium transport in the duct of their eccrine sweat glands. This accounts for the increased concentration of sodium and chloride in the sweat, which for many years has been the main-stay in the diagnosis of this condition [14]. This defect in sodium transport appears to be due to an as yet un-isolated factor in the sweat of patients with CFP [9]. Mangos and McSherry have shown that retrograde perfusion of the rat parotid duct with sweat or saliva from children with CFP results in inhibition of sodium reabsorption [12, 13]. Spock et al. have suggested that the disorganized ciliary beat of rabbit tracheal explants exposed to the sera of patients with CFP may result from a toxic factor altering the transport of electrolytes by the cell [18]. Several other investigators, using different assay systems, have now found evidence for a toxic factor which alters ciliary beat in the plasma of patients with CFP [3, 4, 7].

Balfe, Cole, and Welt have reported abnormalities in sodium transport in erythrocytes of patients with CFP [1]. A decrease in the *pump II* component of Na efflux (*i.e.*, that part of sodium efflux which is inhibited by ethacrynic acid in the presence of maximally inhibiting concentrations of ouabain) in male patients with CFP has been confirmed by Lapey and Gardner [10]. In addition, Horton, Cole, and Bader have reported a decrease in the calcium-activated component of ATPase in patients with CFP [8]. Further studies of ATPase activity in erythrocytes of patients with CFP seemed to be indicated. In the present study, it was decided to study the ouabain-sensitive and ouabain-insensitive components of ATPase in erythrocytes of patients with CFP, and also to determine the effect of plasma from patients with CFP on the ATPase activity of normal erythrocytes.

Methods

Patients used in this study were attending the out-patient clinics of the Montreal Children's Hospital and the Royal Edward Chest Hospital. The 20 patients ranged in age from 7 to 16 years. Their clinical status, as judged by Shwachman scores of 45–90, was moderate to excellent [16]. Fifty-five per cent of the patients were female.

Normal subjects came from a population of healthy young adults. We had previously observed no difference in erythrocyte sodium or potassium, or in ATPase levels between children and adults.

Sodium and potassium in erythrocytes of each patient were measured by washing 3 ml erythrocytes three times with isotonic tetramethylammonium chloride. After the final wash, the erythrocytes were resuspended in a few drops of the wash solution, the hematocrit of the suspension was determined, and the cells were then hemolyzed in lithium diluent. Sodium and potassium contents of the hemolyzed suspension were read on a flame photometer [20], and values were expressed as mEq/liter erythrocytes.

Erythrocyte ATPase was determined on erythrocyte "ghosts" prepared by an osmotic hemolysis technique. Erythrocytes were hemolyzed in a rapidly stirred ice cold solution of 1×10^{-4} M ethylenediaminetetraacetic acid buffered with 5 mM Tris to pH 7.6. After 20 min of stirring, the membranes were separated by centrifugation under refrigeration (20 min at $20,000 \times g$) [21] and washed three times, or until creamy white, with 0.017 M NaCl buffered to pH 7.6 with 5 mM Tris. Three additional washes with 5 mM Tris (pH 7.45) removed all traces of sodium. The membranes were resuspended in the final wash solution, and stored at $-20°$ until used.

ATPase activity of the membranes was assayed in a medium that contained 75 mM Na, 25 mM K, 25 mM Tris (pH 7.45), 1 mM Mg, and 1 mM ATP; these are the ion concentrations which cause maximal activation of the enzyme [6]. The reaction was started with ATP and allowed to proceed for 90 min at 37° before being stopped with 7.5% trichloroacetic acid. The precipitated membranes were spun down, and inorganic phosphorus (Pi) was measured in the supernatant fluid by an autoanalyzer modification of the Lowry Lopez technique [11]. Boiled membrane blanks were run in each experiment. All determinations were performed in duplicate. Dry weight of the membrane suspension was determined on an electrobalance [22] after 24-hr drying in a vacuum oven. Ouabain-sensitive ATPase activity was defined as the difference in activity determined in the presence and absence of 1 mM ouabain [23].

The effect on the ATPase activity of normal erythrocytes of plasma from patients with CFP was determined by incubating 5 ml erythrocytes from control subjects in 5 ml of plasma from patients. The incubating solution contained 100 mg glucose, 7 mg adenine, 13 mg inosine, 0.5 ml 0.1 M sodium phosphate buffer (pH 7.4), 250,000 units penicillin G, and 50 mg streptomycin sulfate. Incubation was continued for 18 hr at 37° in a shaking water bath. Cells were then separated from plasma, "ghosts" were prepared, and ATPase activity was assayed as outlined above.

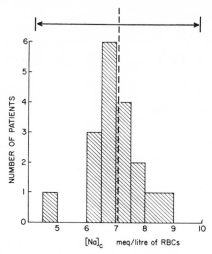

Fig. 1: Sodium concentration in erythrocytes of 20 patients with CFP. The mean erythrocyte sodium concentration in 25 control subjects is indicated by the dotted line. Two standard deviations from this mean are indicated by the horizontal line.

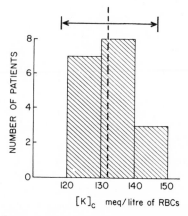

Fig. 2: Potassium concentration in erythrocytes of 20 patients with CFP. The mean erythrocyte potassium concentration in 25 control subjects is indicated by the dotted line. Two standard deviations from this mean are indicated by the horizontal line.

The concentration of sodium in the erythrocytes of 20 patients with CFP fell within our normal range of 4.4–9.8 mEq Na/liter erythrocytes (mean $\pm$ 2 SD). The results are depicted in Figure 1.

Figure 2 shows erythrocyte potassium measurements in the same patients. Again, all values fell within our normal range of 118–147 mEq K/liter erythrocytes (mean $\pm$ 2 SD).

Measurements of ouabain-sensitive ATPase in 20 patients with CFP are shown in Fig. 3. Each patient was paired with a control at the time blood was drawn, and all subsequent steps in the assay were carried out in a tightly paired fashion. There was no consistent change in ouabain-sensitive ATPase activity in erythrocytes of these patients relative to their paired controls. The mean ouabain-sensitive ATPase activity ($\pm$ standard error of the mean) in patients was $10.8 \pm 0.6 \times 10^{-8}$ moles Pi/mg dry weight membrane suspension/hr compared with a value of $10.1 \pm 0.8 \times 10^{-8}$ in the control subjects.

Additional studies revealed no difference in the concentration of Na necessary for half maximal activation of the ouabain-sensitive ATPase activity in patients and control subjects, which suggests that there was no qualitative difference in the ouabain-sensitive component of ATPase in patients and control subjects.

Results of determinations of the ouabain-insensitive component of ATPase in the same patients are presented in Figure 4 and Table I. The mean patient:control subject ratio for ouabain-insensitive activity was 0.90. This decrease in ouabain-insensitive ATPase activity (8.4 ± 0.5 *versus* $9.4 \pm 1.0 \times 10^{-8}$ moles Pi/mg dry weight membrane suspension/hr) was statistically significant ($P < 0.005$) when analyzed with a paired value Student's t test (averaging values for two patients and comparing this with the value for the control subject).

In the determination of the effect of plasma from patients with CFP on the ATPase activity of normal erythrocytes, two series of experiments were performed. In the control series, erythrocytes from normal subjects were divided into two aliquots; one aliquot was incuabated in its own plasma, the other in the plasm-

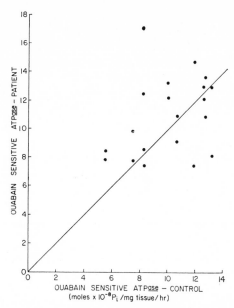

Fig. 3: Comparison of ouabain-sensitive ATPase activity in membranes of erythrocytes from 20 patients with CFP and from paired control subjects. See text for details of assay. The straight line indicates the theoretical line of identity between patient and control.

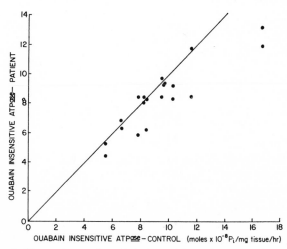

Fig. 4: Comparison of ouabain-insensitive ATPase activity in membranes of erythrocytes from 20 patients with CFP and from paired control subjects.

Table I. Ouabain-insensitive ATPase activity in patients with cystic fibrosis of the pancreas[1]

Control subjects	Patients	
8.4	8.3	6.2
10.3	9.2	8.3
6.6	6.8	6.3
5.5	5.2	4.4
7.8	8.4	5.8
16.7	13.2	11.9
11.6	11.7	8.5
9.6	9.2	9.2
8.2	8.4	8.1
9.5	9.7	8.4
Mean 9.4 ± 1.0	8.4 ± 0.5	

[1] Activity is expressed as moles $\times 10^{-8}$ inorganic phosphorus per milligram tissue per hour.

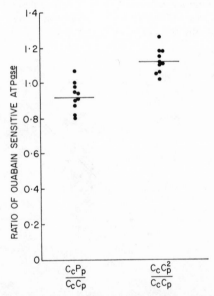

Fig. 5: Ouabain-sensitive ATPase activity of normal erythrocytes after incubation in plasma of: *left:* patient with CFP, and *right:* plasma of another healthy control subject. $C_c P_p$: activity of control cells incubated in patients' plasma. $C_c C_p$: activity of same control cells incubated in own plasma. $C_c C_p^2$: activity of control cells incubated in plasma of another control subject.

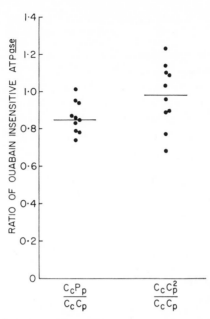

Fig. 6: Ouabain-insensitive ATPase activity of normal erythro-cytes after incubation in plasma of: *left:* patient with CFP, and *right:* another healthy control subject. C_cP_p: activity of control cells incubated in patients' plasma. C_cC_p: activity of same control cells incubated in own plasma. $C_cC_p^2$: activity of control cells incubated in plasma of another control subject.

of another healthy control subject. After incubation, ghosts were prepared and ATPase activity was assayed. Results are expressed as the ratio of ATPase activity of control cells incubated in the plasma of another healthy control subject to that of control cells incubated in their own plasma. For the control series of experiments this ratio was 0.98 for ouabain-insensitive ATPase and 1.12 for ouabain-sensitive ATPase. (See right side of Figures 5 and 6.) This augmentation of ouabain-sensitive ATPase activity following incubation of erythrocytes in foreign plasma has been noted previously [2, 5].

In the second series of experiments, erythrocytes from normal control subjects were divided into 2 aliquots; one was incubated in its own plasma, whereas the other was incubated in fresh plasma from a patient with CFP. After incubation, ghosts were prepared and ATPase activity was assayed. Results are expressed as the ratio of the ATPase activity of control cells incu-bated in the plasma of a patient with CFP to that of

control cells incubated in their own plasma. For ouabain-sensitive ATPase activity, this ratio was 0.92, a
ratio which was significantly different from 1.00 ($P <$
0.01) and significantly different from the ratio for our
control series ($P < 0.001$). These differences retained
the same degree of statistical significance when analyzed
by nonparametric statistics (rank sum test of Wilcoxon).
Thus, it can be concluded that plasma from patients
with CFP is capable of inducing a statistically significant decrease in the ouabain-sensitive ATPase activity
of normal erythrocytes after 18 hr of incubation at 37°.

The effect of plasma from patients with CFP on the
ouabain-insensitive component of ATPase of normal
erythrocytes is shown on the left in Fig. 6. The activity
ratio (*vide supra*) of 0.85 was less than the same ratio for
the control series (on the right in Fig. 6), but the difference between the two ratios was not statistically
significant.

Discussion

In the present series of experiments, we have found no
abnormalities in the ouabain-sensitive component of the
ATP-hydrolyzing enzyme system in erythrocyte membranes of patients with CFP. This finding is in agreement with results reported by Horton, Cole and Bader
[8] and by Besley and Patrick [2]. There is a close relation between the ouabain-sensitive ATP-hydrolyzing
enzyme system in the erythrocyte membrane and active
transport of sodium by the erythrocyte [17]. Thus our
finding of normal ouabain-sensitive ATPase in this
series of patients with CFP is also in agreement with the
recent studies of Lapey and Gardner [10]. Our finding
of normal concentrations of sodium and potassium in
erythrocytes of patients with CFP provides further evidence that the erythrocyte "Na pump" is normal in
these patients.

Although these patients with CFP did not have a decrease in the ouabain-sensitive component of ATPase
in erythrocyte membranes, their plasma was capable of
inducing such a defect in normal erythrocytes. This
finding suggests that erythrocytes in patients with CFP
were able to cope with a toxic factor which was capable
of inducing an ATPase defect in normal cells.

Several investigators have reported evidence for a factor or factors in the plasma, sweat, and saliva of patients with CFP which affect various aspects of sodium transport [3, 9, 14]. Spock *et al.* suggested in 1967 that a macromolecule in the serum of patients with CFP might alter the transport of electrolytes by the cell, thereby producing changes in the action potential within the cell and resulting in a disorganized ciliary beat [18]. One manifestation of the action of such a molecule may be a decrease in the ouabain-sensitive ATPase activity of normal erythrocytes when they are incubated in plasma which contains this molecule.

A decrease in the ouabain-insensitive component of ATPase activity in erythrocytes of patients with CFP has not been previously reported, and its physiological significance is not immediately apparent. This component of ATPase is not involved with active sodium transport by the erythrocyte. Horton *et al.* have reported a decrease, in patients with CFP, of a component of ATPase which requires 3×10^{-4} M calcium for activation, and which is thought to be involved in calcium transport by the erythrocyte membrane [8]. It is possible that this decrease in calcium-activated ATPase may be related to the decrease in the ouabain-insensitive component of ATPase which we have observed.

There is a statistically significant decrease in the mean ouabain-insensitive ATPase activity of the 20 patients whom we have studied. However, it is evident from Figure 4 that all patients do not show this decrease. Since there are marked differences in the severity and symptomatology of CFP, that reflects, at least in part, the genetic heterogeneity of this disease [19], it is not surprising that studies of membrane transport show a similar lack of uniformity.

Summary and Conclusions

Abnormalities in various components of the ATP-hydrolyzing enzyme system in the erythrocyte membrane have been found in patients with CFP. We have found a mean decrease of 10% in the ouabain-insensitive component of ATPase activity in 20 patients with CFP.

The plasma of patients with CFP contains a toxic

factor which causes a decrease in the ouabain-sensitive ATPase activity of normal erythrocytes following 18 hr of incubation in plasma from patients with CFP. The patients themselves show no decrease in ouabain-sensitive ATPase activity in their erythrocytes, and the concentrations of sodium and potassium in their erythrocytes are normal; this suggests that the sodium pump in their erythrocytes is in some way protected from this toxic factor in their plasma.

References and Notes

1. BALFE, J. W., COLE, C., AND WELT, L. G.: Red cell transport defect in patients with cystic fibrosis and in their parents. Science, *162:* 689 (1968).
2. BESLEY, G. T. N., AND PATRICK, A. D.: The effect of cystic fibrosis plasma and saliva on enzyme systems of cell membranes. Proc. 5th Intern. Cystic Fibrosis Conf., p. 14. (Cystic Fibrosis Research Trust, London, 1969).
3. BESLEY, G. T. N., PATRICK, A. D., AND NORMON, A. P.: Inhibition of the mobility of gill cilia of Deissensia by plasma of cystic fibrosis patients and their parents. J. Med. Genet., *6:* 281 (1969).
4. BOWMAN, B. H., McCOMBS, M. L., AND LOCKHART, L. H.: Cystic fibrosis: characterization of inhibition to ciliary action in oyster gills. Science, *167:* 869 (1970).
5. COLE, C. H., BALFE, J. W., AND WELT, L. G.: Induction of a ouabain-sensitive ATPase defect by uremic plasma. Trans. Ass. Amer. Physicians Philadelphia, *31:* 213 (1968).
6. COLE, C. H., AND DIRKS, J.: A comparison of Na^+ activation of ATPase in the red cells, renal cortex and renal medulla. Can. J. Physiol. Pharmacol., *49:* 63 (1971).
7. CRAWFURD, M. D'A.: Experience of the cilia test for a factor in the serum of patients and carriers of cystic fibrosis. Proc. 5th Intern. Cystic Fibrosis Conf., *42* (1969).
8. HORTON, C. R., COLE, W. Q., AND BADER, H.: Decreased Ca transport ATPase in cystic fibrosis erythrocytes. Biochem. Biophys. Res. Commun., *40:* 505 (1970).
9. KAISER, D., DRACK, E., AND ROSSI, E.: Inhibitions of net sodium transport in single sweat islands by sweat of patients with cystic fibrosis of the pancreas. Pediat. Res., *5:* 167 (1971).
10. LAPEY, A., AND GARDNER, J. D.: Abnormal erythrocyte sodium transport in cystic fibrosis. Abstr. Amer. Pediat. Soc., p. 100 (1970).
11. LOWRY, O. H., AND LOPEZ, J. A.: The determination of inorganic phosphate in the presence of labile phosphate esters. J. Biol. Chem., *162:* 421 (1946).
12. MANGOS, J. A., AND McSHERRY, N. R.: A sodium transport inhibitory factor in the saliva of patients with cystic fibrosis of the pancreas. Pediat. Res., *1:* 436 (1967).

13. MANGOS, J. A., AND McSHERRY, N. R.: Sodium transport: inhibitory factor in sweat of patients with cystic fibrosis. Science, *158:* 135 (1967).

14. SANT'AGNESE, P. A., AND TALAMO, R. C.: Pathogenesis and physiopathology of cystic fibrosis of the pancreas. New Engl. J. Med., *277:* 1344 (1967).

15. SATO, K., AND DOBSON, R. L.: Enzymatic basis for the active transport of Na in the duct and secretory portion of the eccrine sweat gland. J. Invest. Dermatol., *55:* 53 (1970).

16. SHWACHMAN, H.: Long term study of 105 patients with cystic fibrosis. Amer. J. Dis. Child., *96:* 6 (1958).

17. Skou, J. C.: Enzymatic basis for active transport of Na^+ and K^+. Physiol. Rev., *45:* 596 (1965).

18. SPOCK, A., HEICK, H. M. C., CRESS, H., AND LOGAN, W. S.: Abnormal serum factor in patients with cystic fibrosis of the pancreas. Pediat. Res., *1:* 173 (1967).

19. WANG, CHUN-I.: Natural variance of cystic fibrosis. Cystic Fibrosis Club Abstracts, p. 5, April 1971.

20. Instrumentation Laboratory, Lexington, Mass.

21. International Equipment Co., Needham Heights, Mass.

22. Cahn Division, Ventron Instruments Corporation, Paramount, Calif.

23. Ouabain octahydrate, Sigma Chemical Company, St. Louis, Mo.

24. The use of human volunteers reported in this paper was reviewed by an ethics committee of McGill University and found acceptable. Informed consent was received from the parents of the children involved.

25. Grateful acknowledgment is made to Mrs. Mary Pan for her excellent technical assistance. The authors wish to thank Dr. Mimi Belmonte for making available the patients from the Montreal Children's Hospital who were used in this study.

The inhibition of ciliary activity in tracheal organ cultures by sera from children with cystic fibrosis and control subjects

James D. Cherry, M.D., Vernon J. Roden, B.S., Anthony J. Rejent, M.D., and Robert W. Dorner, Ph.D.

I n 1967, Spock and associates[1] reported that sera from patients with cystic fibrosis caused disorganized ciliary rhythm in explants of rabbit tracheal tissue. They also noted that sera from parents of children with cystic fibrosis were ciliotoxic. More recently similar findings have been observed in oyster and freshwater mussel gill organ culture preparations.[2, 3]

These reports suggest that large-scale screening for persons who are heterozygous for cystic fibrosis could be possible. However, the culture systems so far described

Supported in part by the Cardinal Glennon Memorial Research Fund and a grant from the National Cystic Fibrosis Research Foundation.

Presented in part to the Cystic Fibrosis Club, Atlantic City, N. J., April 28, 1971.

would appear to be somewhat difficult to prepare, suffer from geographic and seasonal limitations, and be hard to evaluate quantitatively. Recently a chicken embryo tracheal organ culture system has been described which, in addition to allowing large-quantity production, can be accurately accessed for ciliary activity quantitatively.[4, 5] It would seem that this system might be useful in the study of cystic fibrosis. This communication presents the results of our trials with sera from cystic fibrosis patients and control subjects in chicken tracheal organ cultures, as well as similarly prepared rabbit tracheal preparations.

MATERIALS AND METHODS

Study subjects. Sera were obtained from children with cystic fibrosis, confirmed by clinical findings and elevated concentrations of chloride in the sweat, and from healthy control subjects.

Serum specimens. Blood specimens were collected with plastic syringes and discharged into screw-capped tissue culture tubes. The specimens were placed at 4° C., allowed to clot, and the serum was separated by centrifugation at 800g for 10 minutes. Serum was stored at 4° C. until used—usually within one week. Selected sera were heated at 56° C. for 30 minutes, or treated for one hour with 25 per cent acid-washed kaolin.

Organ cultures. The method of preparation of chicken embryo tracheal organ cultures has been previously described.[4] In brief, tracheal ring sections 0.5 to 1 mm. in thickness were cut from embryos that were 19 to 20 days old and placed in screw-capped tissue culture tubes containing 1 ml. of Eagles basal medium (each milliliter contained penicillin G, 100 units; streptomycin, 100 μg; and amphotericin B, 0.25 μg). The ring sections were allowed to adhere to the sides of the tubes and were incubated on a roller drum (15 revolutions per hour) at 35° C.

Utilizing similar techniques, tracheal ring cultures were also prepared from New Zealand–flemish white rabbits that were 2 weeks old. All studies were performed on cultures that were less than 10 days old.

Ciliary activity. Two experimental methods were employed. In the first, the sera to be evaluated were added directly to the tracheal ring containing tubes and examined and evaluated as previously described.[4] In brief, ciliary activity was graded as to its extent as a percentage and also as to its vigor of movement based on an arbitrary scale from 0 to 6+. In previous studies with mycoplasmas, this technique was sensitive and reproducible.[4, 5]

The second, short-term experiments, were performed in either flat-bottomed welled culture slides (Unitron Instrument Co.) or flat-bottomed plastic trays (Linbro Chemical Co., Inc.). In these experiments, rings were removed from the roller culture tubes and placed in the wells. The test serum was added directly to the ring containing well in a volume sufficient to cover the tracheal section. Ciliary activity was observed with an inverted microscope at ×150 magnification. Grading was similar to that used in tube culture preparations, except that in the flat wells ciliary activity frequently could not be visualized throughout the section. In these instances, the percentage of activity was determined on the basis of activity at a particular time compared with that present at the onset of the experiment.

Fractionation of serum. Serum was separated by gel filtration on a Sephadex G-200 column in 0.1M acetate buffer, pH 4. The protein peaks collected, which will be referred to as γM, γG, and albumin fractions according to their chief constituents, were concentrated by negative pressure dialysis, dialyzed against medium 199, and diluted to the original concentration in the same medium.

Dialysis study. Chicken tracheal rings were placed in both halves of a chamber (Technilab Mod. Fl.) separated by a cellulose dialysis membrane. Heat-inactivated serum was introduced into one side and unheated serum from the same subject was added to the other side of the chamber.

Histology. Tracheal ring sections were fixed in gluteraldehyde at 4° C. for 1 hour, washed in buffer, sectioned, and stained with hematoxylin and eosin.

RESULTS

Studies in roller tubes. The sera from 4 children with cystic fibrosis and from 7 control subjects were used in multiple comparative studies in roller tube cultures containing chicken tracheal rings. The results of 5 experiments are recorded in Table I. As can be seen, there is no difference in adverse effect between sera from cystic fibrosis patients and those from normal subjects. All untreated sera in a concentration of 1:24 or greater were ciliotoxic. The toxic factor would appear to be heat labile, as heated serum (56° C. for 30 minutes) at a 1:24 dilution had no adverse effect. In Fig. 1, Experiment 2 is presented in detail. Reduc-

Table I. Ciliary inhibition by serum from cystic fibrosis patients compared with serum from control subjects

Experiment*	Category	No. of subjects	Concentration of serum in medium	Time for 50% reduction of ciliary vigor
1	CF	2	1:6	< 4 hr.
	Control	2	1:6	< 4 hr.
2	CF	1	1:6	45 min.
			1:24	34 hr.
	Control	1	1:6	27 min.
			1:24	48 hr.
3	CF	3	1:24†	>144 hr.
	Control	2	1:24†	>144 hr.
4	CF	3	1:60	> 63 hr.
	Control	2	1:60	> 63 hr.
5	CF	2	1:20, 1:180, 1:240	> 92 hr.
	Control	2	1:20, 1:180, 1:240	> 92 hr.

*In Experiments 1, 3, and 4, five culture tubes were used for each factor investigated; in Experiments 2 and 5, 2 and 3 culture tubes, respectively, were used.

†Serum inactivated (56° C. for 30 minutes).

tion in both vigor and per cent activity differs with serum concentration, but not between the cystic fibrosis and normal sera.

Studies in wells. In an initial experiment, undiluted sera from 9 children with cystic fibrosis and 9 sera from control subjects were studied in chicken tracheal preparations. The mean time of 50 per cent reduction in ciliary vigor occurred in 17.7 minutes in the control serum bathed cultures and 22.4 minutes in those bathed with cystic fibrosis serum. All sera were markedly ciliotoxic, and there was no consistent difference between cystic fibrosis and control sera.

A similar but blind controlled study was conducted, in which the sera from 4 children with cystic fibrosis and from 4 control subjects were investigated. All sera were studied in quadruplicate and the results are recorded in Fig. 2. All sera were ciliotoxic and there is no significant difference between the cilia-stopping effect of cystic fibrosis sera and control sera. Disorganized ciliary rhythm is an integral part of the observed toxicity and is similar in the cystic fibrosis and control serum exposed cultures. Following heat treatment, all sera, both cystic fibrosis and control, were no longer ciliotoxic. A similar blind trial was performed using rabbit

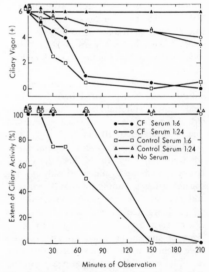

Fig. 1. Cilia-stopping effect of serum from a cystic fibrosis patient compared with serum from a control subject (Experiment 2, Table I).

tracheal ring sections. In this experiment, sera from 3 children with cystic fibrosis were compared with those from 3 control subjects. All sera were ciliotoxic and there

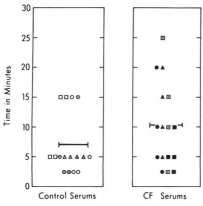

Fig. 2. Time of 50 per cent reduction of ciliary vigor by sera from 4 cystic fibrosis patients compared with sera from 4 control subjects. Studies done blind with 4 trials per serum. (Each symbol represents serum from one patient or control subject.)

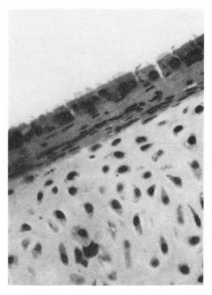

Fig. 3. Rabbit tracheal ring section which was incubated for 2 hours with heat-inactivated control serum.

was no difference in toxicity noted between sera from cystic fibrosis patients and those from control subjects.

To discover the nature of the ciliotoxic factor, further studies were performed. Treatment of serum with 25 per cent acid washed kaolin removed the toxic factor.

In three experiments, the effect on ciliary vigor of the albumin, γG, and γM serum fractions was compared with that of whole serum. In all experiments, the whole serum was rapidly ciliotoxic whereas none of the fractions displayed toxicity. These results would suggest that the toxic factor was either lost on the column or during dialysis or was inactivated during the separation and concentration procedures. In an attempt to see if the factor was lost during dialysis, whole serum was diluted, reconcentrated, and dialyzed against medium 199 in a manner similar to the serum fraction preparations. Although the dialyzed serum lost some toxic activity as compared to a nondialyzed control serum, it was still markedly toxic causing 50 per cent reduction in ciliary vigor within 45 minutes.

Dialysis study. In a further attempt to see

if the toxic factor were dialyzable, chicken tracheal rings were placed in both halves of a chamber, separated by a cellulose dialysis membrane. Heat-inactivated serum from a control subject was introduced into one side and unheated serum from the same control subject was added to the other side of the chamber. The ring in the normal serum had lost all its activity at one hour, whereas the ring in the heat-inactivated serum was still active at 20 hours.

Histology. Fig. 3 shows a rabbit tracheal section incubated for 2 hours with heat-inactivated control serum. As can be seen, the epithelial layer is intact. In contrast, the epithelial surfaces of sections exposed for 30 minutes to both untreated cystic fibrosis and control sera showed marked destruction with eosinophilic degeneration of the cytoplasm. Figs. 4 and 5 compare sections exposed to control and cystic fibrosis serum. There is no apparent difference in pathology between the two.

47

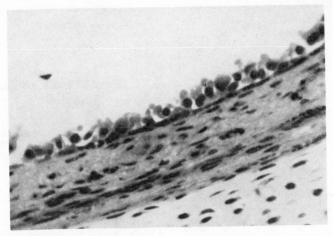

Fig. 4. Rabbit tracheal ring section which was incubated for 30 minutes with untreated control serum. Note marked destruction of the epithelial cells.

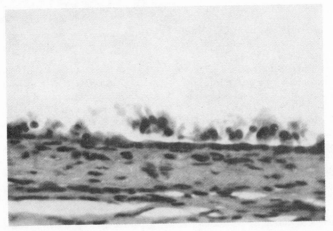

Fig. 5. Rabbit tracheal ring section which was incubated for 30 minutes with untreated cystic fibrosis serum. Note similar appearance to Fig. 4.

DISCUSSION

The present studies were undertaken with the hope that a simple, large-scale surveillance method for the detection of persons with heterozygocity for cystic fibrosis could be developed. The reports of other investigators predicted the success of such a study.[1-3] Although the methods were different, it is hard to reconcile the differences in findings of the present study with the previously reported study which employed rabbit tracheal tissue.[1]

In the present study, all undiluted sera tested were highly toxic to the ciliated epithelia of both rabbit and chicken tracheal organ cultures. The serum ciliotoxic factor was found to be heat labile, nondialyzable, removable by kaolin, and was lost during Sephadex G-200 gel filtration.

We are grateful to Robert Smith, Shafique Ahmad, M.D., Miriam Wiese, and Cleo Hollinshed for their assistance.

REFERENCES

1. Spock, A., Heick, H. M. C., Cress, H., and Logan, W. S.: Abnormal serum factor in patients with cystic fibrosis of the pancreas, Pediatr. Res. 1: 173, 1967.
2. Bowman, B. H., Lockhart, L. H., and McCombs, M. L.: Oyster ciliary inhibition by cystic fibrosis factor, Science 164: 325, 1969.
3. Besley, G. T. N., Patrick, A. D., and Norman, A. P.: Inhibition of the motility of gill cilia of Dreissensia by plasma of cystic fibrosis patients and their parents, J. Med. Genet. 6: 278, 1969.
4. Cherry, J. D., and Taylor-Robinson, D.: Large-quantity production of chicken embryo tracheal organ cultures and use in virus and mycoplasma studies, Appl. Microbiol. 19: 658, 1970.
5. Cherry, J. D., and Taylor-Robinson, D.: Growth and pathogenesis of Mycoplasma mycoides var. capri in chicken embryo tracheal organ cultures, Infect. Immunity 2: 431, 1970.

Opsonic Defect in Patients
with Cystic Fibrosis of the Pancreas

W. D. BIGGAR, B. HOLMES, AND R. A. GOOD

Cystic fibrosis of the pancreas (CFP) is one of the most common inborn errors of metabolism. Frequent manifestations of the disease in children include pancreatic malfunction, an inability to secrete hypotonic sweat normally, and recurrent and chronic pulmonary infections leading to progressive pulmonary insufficiency. The high incidence of morbidity and mortality in CFP is primarily due to the pulmonary component of this disease. Impaired mucociliary clearance of pulmonary debris, chronic endobronchial infection, and severe progressive pulmonary insufficiency characterize the pulmonary pathology. Spock *et al.* (1) described a serum factor present in CFP patients which disrupted the normal rhythmic beating of the cilia in explants of rabbit tracheal epithelium. A similar effect was observed when a nasal polyp that had been excised from a CFP patient was exposed to CFP serum. It can be postulated that this inhibitory factor induces ciliary dyskinesis along the patient's respiratory tract epithelium and disrupts the mucociliary transport system. Impaired mucociliary flow would result in the accumulation of secretions, obstruction of small airways, and the establishment of a suitable environment for bacterial growth.

To date, no immune deficiency has been found in children with CFP. They have normal or elevated quantities of serum and secretory immunoglobulins (2–5) and are capable of producing specific antibody in response to bacterial infection (6).

Abbreviations: CFP, cystic fibrosis of the pancreas; PMN, polymorphonuclear leukocytes; HBSS, Hanks' balanced salt solution.

The organisms cultured from the sputum of CFP patients vary considerably, but the significance of *Pseudomonas aeruginosa* as a pathogen has become apparent (7–9). The successful establishment of this organism as a pathogen may be attributed, at least in part, to the suppression of other bacterial species by antibiotic therapy.

The following study was undertaken to examine the capacity of CFP patients to produce serum factors which promote phagocytosis of Pseudomonas. To this end patients' sera were examined in phagocytosis assays that used blood polymorphonuclear leukocytes (PMN) and rabbit alveolar macrophages.

MATERIALS AND METHODS

Selection of patients

Nine children who regularly attend the cystic fibrosis clinic at the University of Minnesota were studied. The age range was from 6 to 15 years. All patients had an abnormal content of sweat electrolytes and had the characteristic pulmonary manifestations of CFP. In addition, 10 patients were studied who had primary deficiences of humoral immunity alone or in association with deficiences of cellular immunity. Their ages ranged from 8 months to 16 years. Seven of the 10 patients were examined prior to initiation of therapy. Control subjects, aged 4–16 years, were nonhospitalized healthy children who had no history of recurrent sinopulmonary infections.

Polymorphonuclear leukocyte function

Phagocytic capacities of human PMN were determined by the Maalφe method (10) with the modifications described by Cohn and Morse (11) and Hirsch and Strauss (12).

Human peripheral leukocytes were prepared by dextran sedimentation of heparinized venous blood. 10 ml of blood containing 1 mg of heparin was mixed with 2 ml of 6% dextran in saline and incubated at room temperature for 1 hour. The plasma—containing leukocytes, platelets, and few erythrocytes—was withdrawn. The leukocytes were sedimented by centrifugation at $200 \times g$ and washed with heparinized saline. The leukocytes were centrifuged, washed again, and resuspended in Hanks' balanced salt solution (HBSS) (Microbiological Assoc., Bethesda, Md.) to give a concentration of 10×10^6 PMN/ml.

Pseudomonas aerugenosa was obtained from the Diagnostic Laboratory of the University of Minnesota. Organisms were prepared by an overnight incubation in trypticase soy broth in a water-bath shaker at 37°C. The bacteria were collected by centrifugation for 10 min at $1700 \times g$ and resuspended in appropriate dilutions to provide $5–10 \times 10^6$ cells/ml in the stationary growth phase. Sera from patients and controls were

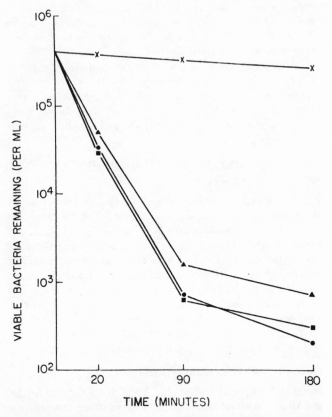

FIG. 1. Viable bacterial counts after incubation for 20, 90, and
180 min with control polymorphonuclear leukocytes (PMN) and
serum from (▲) a normal; (■) a patient with an isolated IgA
deficiency; (✕) a congenital agammaglobulinemic patient; and (●)
a cystic fibrosis patient.

collected from venous blood and used immediately, then
stored in small aliquots at −70°C for future testing.

Phagocytic tests were done in 13 × 75 mm Falcon Plastic
tubes (Falcon Plastics, Division of Bio-Quest Oxnard). Each
tube contained 0.5 ml of leukocyte suspension, 0.1 ml of
bacterial suspension, 0.1 ml of serum, and 0.3 ml of HBSS.
Each assay included patient's serum and control leukocytes or
control serum and control leukocytes.

The tubes for assay of phagocytosis were incubated at 37°C
on a Lab Tech Tilter. 0.1-ml aliquots were removed at 20, 90,
and 180 min. Viable bacteria were quantitated by a standard
dilution-plate technique.

Alveolar macrophage phagocytosis assay

Rabbit alveolar macrophages were obtained by pulmonary lavage according to the method of Myrvik et al. (13). A 1.8- to 2.7-kg New Zealand rabbit was anesthetized with intravenous Nembutal and the lungs and trachea were removed from the thoracic cavity. The lungs were distended with 30 ml of sterile HBSS, massaged, and aspirated with gentle suction. Three lung washings were pooled and centrifuged for 5 min at $200 \times g$. The cell pellet was resuspended in HBSS as a 95% pure macrophage population to contain 4×10^6 cells/ml. More than 95% of the cells isolated exclude trypan blue.

Phagocytic tests were done in Falcon plastic tubes. Each 13×75 mm tube in the phagocytic test contained 0.5 ml of alveolar macrophage suspension, 0.1 ml of a 1:1 dilution of serum in HBSS, 0.1 ml of the suspension of bacteria, and 0.3 ml of HBSS. Each assay included duplicate tests of both test and standardized control sera. The tubes were incubated at 37°C on a Lab Tech Tilter, and 0.1-ml aliquots were removed at 60 and 90 min. Viable bacteria were quantitated by a standard dilution-plate technique.

The phagocytic ratio was calculated as the number of viable extracellular bacteria remaining in the test assay at 90 min divided by the number of viable extracellular bacteria remaining in the control assay.

The method of Mayer (14) was used to determine the serum hemolytic complement activity (C'H50 units).

RESULTS

Fig. 1 shows the results of a typical phagocytosis assay to test the various sera for the promotion of phagocytosis by PMN. Sera from patients with CFP were found to have the same capacity to promote phagocytosis of *Pseudomonas* by PMN as normal control sera. When increasing dilutions of CFP serum were tested, the sera of these patients continued to support phagocytosis of Pseudomonas by PMN as well as or better than control sera of the same dilution. Seven of the ten sera from patients with primary immunological deficiencies failed to promote phagocytosis of Pseudomonas by PMN of normal controls. Two of three patients with immunological deficiencies whose sera promoted normal phagocytosis had isolated severe deficiencies of IgA. The third had mild hypogammaglobulinemia.

Fig. 2 shows the capacity of the various sera to promote phagocytosis of Pseudomonas by alveolar macrophages. For normal sera, the mean phagocytic ratio was 2.8 ± 1.1 (SE). Normal serum heated at 56°C for 30 min did not promote phagocytosis. Similarly, no phagocytosis occurred when serum was decomplemented by antigen–antibody complexes. Six of

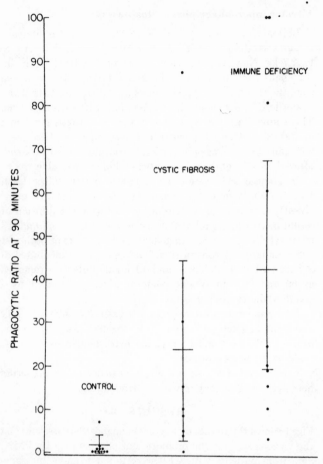

Fig. 2. Phagocytic ratio of alveolar macrophage phagocytosis by normal serum and by sera from patients with cystic fibrosis of the pancreas and primary immunological deficiencies. The phagocytic ratio was calculated as the number of viable extracellular bacteria remaining in the test assay at 90 min divided by the number of viable extracellular bacteria remaining in the control assay.

the nine sera from CFP patients showed a marked deficiency in the promotion of phagocytosis. Quantitative immunoglobulin determinations showed normal or elevated levels of immunoglobulins and normal total serum hemolytic complement activity. With increasing concentrations of CFP serum, the capacity to promote phagocytosis improved. Preliminary results indicate that approximately four times the concentration of CFP serum is required for normal phagocytosis.

54

Nine of ten sera from immune deficiency patients failed to promote phagocytosis. Two of these nine patients had isolated deficiences of serum IgA (<6 mg/100 ml), four had severe hypogammaglobulinemia, and three had severe combined dual system immunodeficiencies. The tenth patient, whose serum supported phagocytosis normally, had mild hypogammaglobulinemia and infrequent pulmonary infections.

DISCUSSION

Phagocytosis of bacteria is a complex series of events. This includes the interaction of the bacterium with humoral factors (heat-stable and heat-labile opsonins), attraction and adherence to the phagocyte, and finally, ingestion. Chemical and physical environmental factors greatly influence the outcome of the interaction between a microorganism and the phagocyte. Serum factors, critical in influencing the efficiency of phagocytosis, include specific antibody, complement, and other less well-defined components. These are capable of interacting with the surface of bacteria to change its properties (12, 15). In addition, some serum antibodies (cytophilic antibodies) are capable of "fixing" to cells and influencing the specificity and efficiency of that cell's participation in an immune response (16). The rate and the efficiency of the phagocytic process is also influenced by temperature, pH, and divalent cation concentration of the supporting milieu (17, 18).

Malfunction within this complex and dynamic process of phagocytosis may result in deficiences of phagocytosis and an increased susceptibility to infection.

Recently, a group of clinical disorders characterized by abnormalities of phagocytosis and an increased susceptibility to infection have been described. The patients, as distinct from those with the usual immune deficiency syndromes, appear to have a normal capacity to execute humoral and cellular immune responses, but have a failure of the normal inflammatory process. Since chronic granulomatous disease was first clearly defined as a failure of normal killing of certain bacteria by PMN (19), several additional defects in the normal processing of microorganisms by PMN have been described. These syndromes include opsonic deficiencies (20, 21), complement abnormalities (22), and functional abnormalities of the PMN (23–25). None of the serum defects thus far described has been studied with the alveolar macrophage. If we consider comparative studies of monocytes and neutrophils (26), differences in serum factor requirements might also be expected when alveolar macrophages are compared to PMN.

The alveolar macrophage resides in the lung and there represents a primary defense mechanism against a wide variety of stimuli. The environment of the lung is in many ways unique and differs considerably from the environment of the circulating PMN and the peritoneal macrophage. Furthermore, the alveolar macrophage is metabolically and functionally different from the blood PMN and the peritoneal macrophage (27).

Our studies of the phagocytosis of Pseudomonas by the alveolar macrophage indicate that, as with the PMN, both immunoglobulin and complement are required. Neither cell type effectively phagocytizes Pseudomonas in decomplemented serum or sera from patients with primary immunoglobulin deficiencies.

Sera from CFP patients contain normal quantities of immunoglobulin and hemolytic complement and support normal phagocytosis of Pseudomonas by blood PMN. Furthermore, with increasing dilutions, sera from CFP patients promote phagocytosis as well as or better than normal serum. Sera of two patients with severe deficiencies of serum IgA (<6 mg/100 ml) but normal quantities of IgG and IgM were also capable of promoting phagocytosis of Pseudomonas by PMN from controls. Patients with primary immunodeficiency diseases, on the other hand, showed little or no opsonic activity (28).

In contrast, six of nine sera from CFP patients failed to support phagocytosis of Pseudomonas by rabbit alveolar macrophages. That this failure to support phagocytosis is due to a deficiency and not to an inhibitor is evidenced by the capacity of the abnormal serum to correct the phagocytic defect when the concentration used in the test assay is increased. As was observed with PMN, serum from immunodeficiency patients, heat-inactivated serum, or serum previously treated with antigen–antibody complexes failed to promote phagocytosis. Serum from the IgA-deficient patients also failed to support phagocytosis.

The role of IgA in promoting phagocytosis by alveolar macrophages is unknown. IgA does not ordinarily fix complement (29) and does not appear to be essential for phagocytosis by the PMN. The alveolar macrophage functions in a unique milieu, and is in contact with secretions of which IgA is the primary immunoglobulin. It is possible that the alveolar macrophage has different opsonic requirements, with IgA playing a major role in their capacity to phagocytize Pseudomonas.

The requirement for complement in this assay is, of course, difficult to explain if IgA is the only immunoglobulin involved. IgG and (or) IgM and complement, together with IgA, may be required for completely normal phagocytosis. On the other hand, the requirement for complement appears to be absolute and indicates that a complement-fixing antibody is of primary importance. An analysis of alternative pathways for the activation of the later components of complement may resolve the apparent contradiction. Our studies raise the possibility that the defect observed in CFP patients represents a failure to produce adequate IgA antibodies specific for Pseudomonas and is important in the pathogenesis of the progressive pulmonary disease.

The alveolar macrophage phagocytosis assay described here has revealed that six out of nine sera from CFP fail to support normal phagocytosis of Pseudomonas. Since IgA appears to be important in this assay of phagocytosis, it is postulated that CFP patients may have a quantitative and (or) functional defect of IgA antibodies specific for Pseudomonas. Experiments are in progress to test this hypothesis.

We thank Warren J. Warwick for permission to study his patients and Sue Buron for her excellent technical assistance. This work was carried out in the Pediatric Research Laboratories of the Variety Club Heart Hospital and was supported by The National Foundation-March of Dimes, U.S. Public Health Service (AI-08677, HE-06314 and AI-00798), the American Heart Association (70-771) and the National Science Foundation GIB-16835. W. D. B. is a fellow of the Queen Elizabeth II Canadian Research Fund, B. H. an Established Investigator of the American Heart Aosociation, and R. A. G. an American Legion Memorial Research Professor and Regents' Professor of Pediatrics, Microbiology and Pathology.

1. Spock, A., H. M. C. Heick, H. Cress, and W. S. Logan, *Pediat. Res.*, 1, 173 (1967).
2. Schwartz, R. H., *Amer. J. Dis. Child.*, 111, 408 (1966).
3. Wagstaff, B. W., E. W. Aldour, M. L. Rallison, and D. C. Helner, *Soc. Ped. Res. 36th Annual Meeting* (abstract), p. 67 (1966).
4. South, M. A., W. J. Warwick, F. A. Wollheim, and R. A. Good, *J. Pediat.*, 71, 645 (1967).
5. Martinez-Tello, F. J., D. G. Braun, and W. A. Blanc, *J. Immunol.*, 101, 989 (1968).
6. Burns, M. W., and J. R. May, *Lancet*, 1, 270 (1968).
7. Huang, N. N., E. L. Van Loon, and K. T. Sheng, *J. Pediat.*, 59, 512 (1961).
8. Iacocca, V. F., M. S. Sibinga, and G. J. Barbero, *Amer. J. Dis. Child.*, 106, 315 (1963).
9. Doggett, R. G., G. M. Harrison, R. M. Stillwell, and E. S. Wallis, *J. Pediat.*, 68, 215 (1966).
10. Maaløe, O., Doctoral thesis, Munksgaard, Copenhagen (1946).
11. Cohn, Z. A., and S. I. Morse, *J. Exp. Med.*, 110, 419 (1959).
12. Hirsch, J. C., and B. Strauss, *J. Immunol.*, 92, 145 (1964).
13. Myrvik, Q. N., E. S. Leake, and B. Fariss, *J. Immunol.*, 86, 128 (1961).
14. Mayer, M. M., in *Experimental Immunochemistry*, ed. E. A. Kabat and M. M. Mayer (Charles C Thomas, Springfield, Ill., 1961), pp. 131–240.
15. Rowley, D. *Advan. Immunol.*, 2, 241 (1962).
16. Pearsall, N. N., and R. S. Weiser, in *The Macrophage* (Lea

and Febiger, Philadelphia, 1970), pp. 93–100.
17. Chernew, I., and A. I. Braude, *J. Clin. Invest.*, **41**, 1945 (1962).
18. Mudd, S., M. McCutcheon, and B. Lucke, *Physiol. Rev.*, **14**, 210 (1934).
19. Holmes, B., P. G. Quie, D. B. Windhorst, and R. A. Good. *Lancet* i, 1225 (1966).
20. Forman, M. L., and E. R. Stiehm, *N. Engl. J. Med.*, **281**, 926 (1969).
21. Winkelstein, J. A., and R. H. Drachman, *N. Engl. J. Med.*, **279**, 459 (1968).
22. Miller, M. E., and U. R. Nilsson, *N. Engl. J. Med.*, **282**, 354 (1970).
23. Miller, M. E., F. A. Oski, and M. B. Harris, *Lancet*, i, 665 (1971).
24. Lehrer, R. I., and M. J. Cline, *J. Clin. Invest.*, **48**, 1478 (1969).
25. Ward, P. A., and R. J. Schlegel, *Lancet*, ii, 344 (1969).
26. Douglas, S. D., *Blood*, **35**, 851 (1970).
27. Pearsall, N. N., and R. S. Weiser, in *The Macrophage* (Lea and Febiger, Philadelphia, 1970), pp. 41–56.
28. Williams, R. C., and P. G. Quie, *J. Immunol.*, **106**, 51 (1971).
29. Ishizaka, T., K. Ishizaka, T. Borsos, and H. Rapp, *J. Immunol.*, **97**, 716 (1966).

DISTRIBUTION OF PULMONARY BLOOD FLOW IN CHILDREN WITH CYSTIC FIBROSIS

M. ŠAMÁNEK, J. HOUŠTĚK, V. VÁVROVÁ, C. RUTH and O. ŠNOBL

Pulmonary involvement is responsible for most of the complications and mortality in cystic fibrosis. Since plugging of airways with excessive secretion of mucus is one of the main features of pulmonary pathology it might be expected that, besides close clinical follow-up, ventilatory function studies should be most appropriate in assessment of the severity of pulmonary involvement (4, 8, 9, 12, 21). Unfortunately, in childhood during several critical years spirometric measurements are difficult or impossible for technical reasons. Moreover, these techniques are not able to detect regional differences in lung function. Therefore other methods must have been searched for.

Lung scanning has been extensively used for the evaluation of pulmonary blood flow distribution in different clinical conditions. An attempt to use the measurement of pulmonary blood flow distribution for the assessment of disturbances primarily in ventilation was stimulated by our previous work on ventilation–perfusion relationships (13). The advantage of this method for the studies of regional pulmonary function in children with the obstruction of the airways, including cystic fibrosis, has been documented (6, 14). The present report concerns the regional changes in distribution of pulmonary blood flow and their value for the early detection and follow-up of

pulmonary function abnormalities in cystic fibrosis. Special attention was paid to repeated measurements of pulmonary blood flow distribution in the same patient.

MATERIAL AND METHODS

Thirty lung scans were obtained in 19 children below 6 years of age and in 2 older patients with cystic fibrosis (Table 1). The diagnosis was based on the clinical history and on repeated physical and radiological examinations over a long period. It was confirmed by analysis of the sweat chloride concentration using the method of electrical conductivity (3). Criteria of Shwachman & Kulczycki (17) were used to score the clinical condition of our patients. Body height and weight were expressed in percentiles (18). Chest roentgenograms were obtained by the usual technique in the upright position, with the exception of children younger than 1 year of age, in which the supine position was preferred. The pictures were taken in the maximal inspiration. Respiratory function studies have been performed only in 5 children (case 2, 4, 15, 16, 18) because of the low age of most of our patients, and they are included in the previous report (7). Arterialised capillary blood oxygen tension was measured by the microelektrode of Clark type. The acid–base status of the blood was determined at 37°C by the Astrup equilibration technique (2). Regional blood flow distribution was measured by lung scanning. Macroaggregated human serum albumin (particle size 10 to 75μ) tagged with ^{99m}Tc was injected intravenously in the same position as used for taking X-ray pictures. The isotope dose ranged between 50 and 500 microcuries according to the age of the patient. The total amount of albumin did not reach 0.001 mg/kg body weight. A

Table 1. *Data on patients and results of studies*[a]

Case no.	Name	Sex	Age (y.: mo.)	Height (per-centil)	Weight (per-centil)	Sweat Cl' (mEq/l)	Clinical score	Arterial blood P_{O_2} torr	P_{CO_2} torr	pH	HCO'_3 (mEq/l)
1	P. T.	♂	3: 3	70	50	96.6	85	82	31	7.362	17.1
2	R. D.	♀	5: 9	50	70	102.4	85	73	39	7.386	23.0
3	M. H.	♀	0: 6	40	50	114.4	78	85	36	7.406	22.2
			0: 7	40	50	—	78	—	—	—	—
4	M. V.	♀	11: 7	20	30	100.4	78	102	37	7.450	25.1
			11: 8	20	30	—	78	90	34	7.455	23.5
5	M. M.	♂	1: 5	90	50	103.9	77	90	31	7.419	19.4
6	E. J.	♂	4: 9	10	70	81.7	76	112	28	7.420	17.8
7	A. H.	♂	3: 6	10	20	128.4	73	—	31	7.440	20.0
8	J. P.	♀	4: 9	10	40	104.4	68	—	—	—	—
9	P. H.	♂	3: 10	10	3	124.4	67	103	38	7.456	25.0
10	T. L.	♂	5: 0	3	20	115.4	65	70	37	7.398	22.0
11	P. M.	♂	1: 1	10	10	108.9	64	70	37	7.400	22.3
			2: 2	30	50	—	63	68	37	7.371	20.7
12	H. P.	♀	3: 6	10	3	89.2	63	93	39	7.385	23.0
13	L. B.	♀	1: 8	3	3	116.9	63	90	39	7.412	24.5
14	M. S.	♂	0: 5	70	10	82.6	55	75	49	7.373	28.1
15	M. H.	♂	3: 0	80	20	117.4	55	—	48	7.343	25.3
			4: 7	20	30	—	49	76	51	7.355	28.1
			4: 8	20	30	—	—	—	45	7.409	28.0
16	L. S.	♂	20: 2	90	40	70.2	54	—	—	—	—
			20: 3	90	40	—	54	53	41	7.432	26.9
			20: 4	90	40	—	54	55	40	7.426	25.9
17	D. F.	♀	4: 4	3	10	84.4	51	58	42	7.393	24.8
18	J. H.	♂	5: 11	3	3	120.5	50	100	34	7.442	22.3
			6: 11	5	3	—	46	70	33	7.406	20.3
19	K. M.	♀	4: 5	30	3	115.4	50	80	40	7.458	27.0
			4: 6	30	3	—	45	80	40	7.439	26.1
20	L. M.	♀	2: 1	3	3	101.3	49	77	44	7.388	25.6
			3: 0	3	3	—	52	84	34	7.399	20.2
21	A. D.	♀	1: 0	10	3	91.9	48	83	29	7.448	19.2

[a] Grade: 0 = normal, 1 = slight, 2 = moderate, 3 = marked. Localization: RU, RM, RL = right upper, middle, lower area; LU, LM, LL = left upper, middle, lower area. t = total, p = partial, d = diffuse, c = cystoid.

rectilinear scanner (Pho/Dot, Nuclear Chicago) equipped with 127-hole collimator was used for the detection of the distribution of the macroaggregates. Both X-ray picture and lung scan were usually taken within the shortest possible period of time in the same day.

The evaluation of regional perfusion was done in a similar way as in the chest roentgenograms. Both lungs were divided by the horizontal lines into three even areas not corresponding exactly to the lung lobes. Peribronchial thickening, hyperaeration on roentgenograms, and underperfusion on lung scan was divided according to the intensity into 3 grades. The radioactivity equal to the background activity is called underperfusion of the grade 3 in contrast to the underperfusion of the grade 0, equal to the maximal radioactivity concentration. Partial or total involvement of individual areas indicates the extent of these changes. In 8 patients repeated measurements of regional pulmonary blood flow were performed with an interval ranging from 1 week up to 1 year and 8 months.

RESULTS

Normal distribution of the pulmonary blood flow was detected only in 8 children in our

Chest roentgenogram

Peribronchial thickening		Localized density	Hyperaeration Grade	Lung scan Underperfusion	
Grade	Localization			Grade	Localization
0	—	0	0	0	—
2	RUt, RLt	0	1 d	3	RUp, RMp
1	LLp			2	RUt
1	RUt, LUt	RUt	1 d	0	—
1	RUt, LUt	RUt	1 d	2	RUt
				1	RLp
2	RMp, RLp, LLp	0	1 d	3	LUt
				2	RMp
2	RMt, RLt, LLp	0	2 d	2	LUt, RMp
1	RUt, RLp, LUt	0	0	0	—
1	RUp, RLp	0	0	0	—
1	RUt, RMt, LUt, LMt	0	2 d	1	RUt
2	RUp, RLp, LUp, LLp	0	1 d	0	—
2	RUt, RMt, LUt	0	1 d	1	Multiple
3	Generalized	0	2 d	3	RUp, RMp, LUt
				2	RUt, RLp
1	RLp, LLp	RLp	2 d	3	RUp, RMt
1	RUt, LUt	RLp	3 d	2	RLp, LUp
1	RUp, RLp	0	1 d	1	LUp
2	RLp, LMp	RLp, LMp	1 d	0	—
2	RUt, RMt, RLt, LMt	LMp, RUp	2 d	0	—
3	RMt, RLt, LMt, LLt	RMp, LMp	3 c	2	RUp, LUp
3	RUt, RMt, RLt, LMp, LLt	LLp	2 d	2	RUp, RMp, RLp, LLp
				2	RUp, RMp, RLp, LLp
3	RMt, RLt	0	3 d	3	RUt, LUt
				2	RMp, LMp
3	RMt, RLt	0	3 d	3	RUt, LUt
				2	RMp, LMp
3	RMt, RLt	0	3 d	3	RUt, LUt
				2	RMp, LMp
3	Generalized	RLp, RMp, LLp	2 c	3	RUt
				2	LUp, LLp
3	Generalized	0	3 d	3	RUt, RMp, LUp
				2	LMp
3	Generalized	0	3 d	3	RUt, RMp
				2	LMp
3	Generalized	0	3 c	2	RUp, RMp, RLp, LLp
				2	RUp, RMp, LUt, LMp
2	RUp, RMp, LUp, LMp	RUp, LLp	2 d	0	—
2	RUt, RLp, LLp	0	1 d	0	—
2	RUp, LUp	RLp	1 d	2	RUt

series (Table 1). The most frequent incidence of local changes in perfusion was encountered in the right upper area, followed by the right middle and left upper area (Table 2 and Fig. 1). The combination of partial and total involvement of several areas was usual. Only in 4 children solitary total or partial underperfusion of one area appeared. Marked and moderate changes in perfusion or their combination were most frequent.

By dividing our patients according to the

Table 2. *Regional distribution of underperfusion*

Lung area	Incidence of underperfusion (%)
Right	
Upper	81
Middle	67
Lower	29
Left	
Upper	57
Middle	29
Lower	33

61

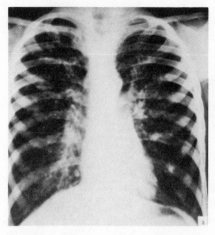
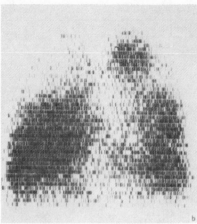

Fig. 1. J. H. (case 18). (a) Chest roentgenogram shows generalized marked peribronchial thickening and diffuse hyperaeration. (b) Lung scan shows most frequent localization of perfusion defects (see Table 1).

clinical scoring method (17) three groups became apparent. Only in 50% of the patients in good clinical condition (case 1–7) normal pulmonary blood flow distribution was revealed (Fig. 2). High frequency of abnormalities in distribution was encountered in the group with mild clinical condition (case 8–13), and in the group with the lowest clinical score (case 14–21). Nevertheless, in the latter group normal distribution pattern was also detected.

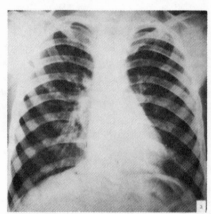
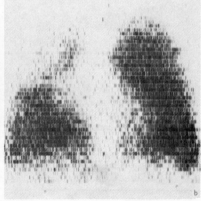

Fig. 2. R. D. (case 2). (a) Chest roentgenogram shows moderate degree of peribronchial thickening, mostly of the right side with diffuse hyperinflation of low degree. (b) Lung scan demonstrates abnormalities in blood flow distribution, not predictable either from clinical or radiological examination.

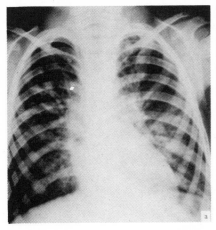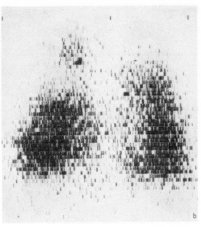

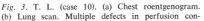

Fig. 3. T. L. (case 10). (a) Chest roentgenogram. (b) Lung scan. Multiple defects in perfusion con-

trasted with the generalized image on chest roentgenogram.

Both, normal and pathological local distribution of pulmonary blood flow was detected in children with the impairment of pulmonary gas exchange indicated by the elevation of P_{CO_2} and by the decrease in P_{O_2} values in arterialised capillary blood. Correlation between the severity of distribution abnormalities and disturbances in gas exchange was not revealed.

Radiological evidence of pulmonary involvement participates in clinical scoring. However, comparison of lung scans with chest roentgenograms alone was necessary for the estimation of the value of both techniques in patients with cystic fibrosis (Table 1). In all but one patient peribronchial thickening of different intensity was evident from the chest roentgenogram. In the majority of cases localization of radiological changes and abnormalities in the distribution of radioactivity correlated only partially. In one third of investigations marked discrepancy was found. Focal changes in density were detected on 11 roentgenograms. Their localization did not agree in 64% of investigations with the localization of perfusion inequalities. On the other hand areas of marked underper-

fusion were revealed by lung scanning in patients without focal changes in X-ray density (Fig. 3).

Repeated scanning was performed in 8 patients. Different pictures of blood flow distribution were obtained in 5 patients (case 3, 11, 15 a, 18, 19). Marked changes in the distribution pattern within an interval shorter than 1 month were revealed in two of them without apparent change of the clinical condition (case 3, 11). In the third child (case 15) the spreading of distribution abnormalities after a longer interval was accompanied by the deterioration of the clinical condition. The change only in the localization of underperfused areas was combined with the lowering of clinical score in two children (case 18, 19).

Unchanged distribution was found three times (case 4, 16, 20) after an interval of 1 month or 1 year, respectively. The discrepancy between stationary pattern of blood flow distribution and changing clinical picture was detected in two patients (case 16, 20). During the first measurement one of them (case 20) was in a fair clinical condition. Surprisingly, lung scan showed marked disturbances in per-

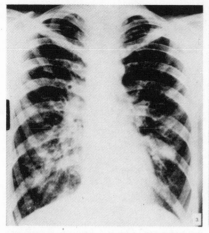

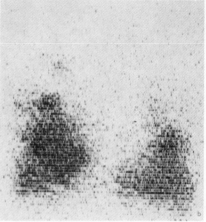

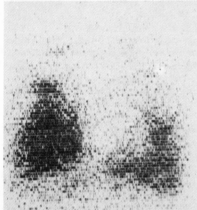

Fig. 4. L. S. (case 16). (a) Chest roentgenogram taken at the same data as the second lung scan shows marked peribronchial thickening and hyperaeration with decreased density in left upper area. (b) and (c) Lung scans recorded with an interval of 10 weeks show identical pattern of blood flow distribution.

fusion (Fig. 4 b). These changes did not improve after the intensive treatment. One week later this patient was admitted to the hospital in respiratory distress due to acute respiratory infection and a small localized left-sided pneumothorax. After the recovery an identical distribution pattern persisted (Fig. 4 c).

DISCUSSION

Lung scanning is believed to be very useful in the diagnosis of pathologic processes involving the pulmonary vascular bed. However, no significant changes in pulmonary arteries and arterioles were found in cystic fibrosis (5). The high incidence of the abnormalities in pulmonary blood flow distribution proved in our patients must therefore be caused by another mechanism. This mechanism has not been firmly established yet. It is reasonable to assume that disturbances in the patency of the airways play an important role in evoking secondary changes in perfusion by two principal mechanisms. The obstruction of bronchi and/ or bronchioles is followed by profound changes in the composition of alveolar gas, namely decrease in P_{O_2} and increase in P_{CO_2}. Increase in the airway resistance causes the enhanced respiratory fluctuations of transpulmonary pressure. During expiration alveolar pressure distal to the partial airway obstruction increase considerably (9). Both changes in alveolar gas tension and in intraalveolar pressure elicite local increase in pulmonary vascular resistance and consequently decrease of blood flow in this region (1).

This mechanism was proved to be responsible for the perfusion abnormalities under several conditions leading to the local obstruction of the airways. In acute asthmatic attack marked local defects in perfusion were demonstrated in children with otherwise normal pulmonary blood flow distribution (10, 16). To prove that the obstruction of airways is responsible for the change on lung scan, blood flow distribution was measured after partial bronchial obstruction by unilateral bronchography. Transient perfusion abnormalities were of the same character as during an asthmatic attack (16). The changes in regional perfusion following localized obstruction of the airways were not identical with the changes in regional ventilation (19). On the contrary Gyepes et al. (6) were able to demonstrate the local coincidence of ventilation and perfusion defects. The existence of perfusion disturbances and their variability in our patients favours the participation of mechanism regulating perfusion according to the ventilation in pulmonary pathophysiology of cystic fibrosis.

Open question remains the efficiency of this mechanism in maintaining perfect gas exchange. If the diminution of perfusion matches localy and qualitatively the decrease in ventilation, no disturbance in pulmonary gas exchange would develop. However, the studies of local regulation of ventilation-perfusion ratio have shown some limitations of this mechanism (15, 20). This may explain low ventilation-perfusion ratio revealed in patients with cystic fibrosis (11). Whatever is the efficiency of this mechanism, local inequalities of perfusion in our patients with the obstructive lung disease must have favourable effect on gas exchange. If the lungs were not able to shift blood away from underventilated regions the incidence of abnormal values of arterial gas tension might be expected to be higher.

Roentgenography has been widely used in the assessment of pulmonary involvement in cystic fibrosis. The limitations of this method in detection of local changes in perfusion has been demonstrated by comparison with lung scanning in this study. The lack of correlation between both methods was encountered. The most frequent finding on chest roentgenograms was peribronchial thickening and diffuse hyperaeration. There is no reason to expect changes of this character to be reflected by the local abnormality of perfusion. Localized changes of X-ray density, without regard of their etiology, should manifest themselves as the change in perfusion. This was not the case in the majority of our patients. On the other hand even marked defects in perfusion shown by lung scanning were not revealed by roentgenography. In view of these facts there is no reason to underestimate the value of roentgenography in cystic fibrosis. Its importance is primarily in depicting anatomical pulmonary lesions and its value was documented also in our study. The main advantage of lung scanning is in the detection of regional changes in perfusion i.e. in the detection of a functional abnormality. Our study has shown that both methods are very useful but not interchangeable.

By use of criteria indicated above, three clinical groups of patients were differentiated in our material. The explanation of the lack of exact correlation between the severity of the illness and incidence of the disturbance in perfusion must be searched for in the above mentioned mechanism of development of the perfusion changes. If we accept the assumption that the regional abnormalities in perfusion are secondary to the ventilation disturbances, then the defects in perfusion depend solely on the magnitude and character of the airway obstruction. On the other hand the clinical picture is composed also by many other factors.

Variability in bronchial obstruction is typical for the early stage of pulmonary involvement, whereas fixed changes can be interpreted as permanent disturbance of pulmonary function, signalizing the unfavourable progression of the disease (8). Early detection of dynamics of these functional abnormalities by repeated lung scanning may have considerable implications in the management, especially in the age when lung function studies are not available. Repeated scanning can be used also as one of the indicators of the therapeutical effect. Lung scanning, as a highly reproducible, simple and relatively safe procedure, available in any age offers new possibilities in clinical follow-up of patients with cystic fibrosis and it should be included among other criteria for the assessment of clinical condition and mainly pulmonary involvement in cystic fibrosis.

SUMMARY

Marked abnormalities of pulmonary blood flow distribution were detected in 13 out of 21 children with cystic fibrosis using lung scanning. Underperfusion of different grade was localized most frequently in the right upper area, followed by the right middle and left upper areas. Correlation between clinical condition or impairment of gas exchange and degree of perfusion disturbances was lacking. Abnormal chest roentgenograms were encountered more frequently than the definite disturbances in the distribution of perfusion. On the other hand, even profound defects of perfusion were not revealed by chest roentgenography. Repeated lung scanning might be helpful in the evaluation of the dynamics of pulmonary involvement in cystic fibrosis.

REFERENCES

1. Arborelius, M., Jr: *Respiratory gases and pulmonary blood flow. A bronchospirometric study.* Landby & Lundgren, Malmö 1966.
2. Astrup, P.: A simple electrometric technique for the determination of carbon dioxide tension in blood plasma, total content of carbon dioxide in plasma, and bicarbonate content in separated plasma at a fixed carbon dioxide tension (40 mmHg). *Scand J Clin Lab Invest, 8:* 33, 1956.
3. Bloxsom, A. P.: The electrical conductivity of electrolytes found in the sweat of patients with cystic fibrosis of the pancreas. *Arch Dis Child, 34:* 420, 1959.
4. Cook, C. D., Helliesen, P. J., Kulczycki, L. L., Barrie, H., Friedlander, L., Agathon, S., Harris, G. B. C. & Shwachman, H.: Studies of respiratory physiology in children. II. Lung volumes and mechanics of respiration in 64 patients with cystic fibrosis of the pancreas. *Pediatrics, 24:* 181, 1959.
5. Esterly, J. R. & Oppenheimer, E. H.: Observations in cystic fibrosis of the pancreas. III. Pulmonary lesions. *Johns Hopkins Med J, 122:* 94, 1968.
6. Gyepes, M. E., Bennett, L. R. & Hassakis, P. C.: Regional pulmonary blood flow in cystic fibrosis. *Amer J Roentgen, 106:* 567, 1969.
7. Houštěk, J., Vávrová, V. & Vokáč, Z.: Lung function studies in mucoviscidosis. *Vnitřní Lék, 16:* 449, 1970.
8. Mearns, M. B.: Simple tests of ventilatory capacity in children with cystic fibrosis. *Arch Dis Child 43:* 528, 1968.
9. Mellins, R. B., Levine, O. R., Ingram, R. H., Jr & Fishman, A. P.: Obstructive disease of the airways in cystic fibrosis. *Pediatrics, 41:* 560, 1968.
10. Mishkin, F. & Wagner, H. N., Jr: Regional abnormalities in pulmonary arterial blood flow during acute asthmatic attacks. *Radiology, 88:* 142, 1967.
11. Moss, A. J., Desilets, D. T., Higashino, S. M., Ruttenberg, H. D., Marcano, B. A. & Dooley, R. R.: Intrapulmonary shunts in cystic fibrosis. *Pediatrics, 41:* 438, 1968.
12. Phelan, P. D., Gracey, M., Williams, H. E. & Anderson, C. M.: Ventilatory function in infants with cystic fibrosis. Physiological assessment of inhalation therapy. *Arch Dis Child, 44:* 393, 1969.
13. Šamánek, M. & Aviado, D. M.: Interrelationships between pulmonary blood flow and bronchomotor tone: P_{O_2} and P_{CO_2}. *J Appl Physiol, 22:* 719, 1967.
14. Šamánek, M., Ruth, C., Hloušková, Z., Čopová, M. & Špičák, V.: Pulmonary blood flow distribution in children with obstruction of airways. *Annual Meeting Soc Europ Physiol Clin Respir,* Bochum 1969. In press.
15. Šamánek, M.: Distribution of pulmonary blood flow in patients with abnormal pulmonary pressure and flow. *Progr Resp Research,* Karger, Basel 1970.
16. — Local interrelationships between ventilation and pulmonary blood flow. *J Franc Méd Chir Thorac,* 1969.
17. Shwachman, H. & Kulczycki, L. L.: Long-term study of one hundred and five patients with cystic fibrosis: studies made over a 5–14 year-period. *Amer J Dis Child, 96:* 6, 1958.
18. Stuart, H. C. & Reed, R. B.: Longitudinal studies on child health and development. *Pediatrics, 24:* 875, 1959.

Immunochemical Studies of Cystic Fibrosis Tissues: The Detection of Increased Concentrations of an Antigen which was Identified as C-Reactive Protein[1]

E. L. Greene, S. P. Halbert and J. C. Pallavicini

Cystic fibrosis (CF) is an inherited disease which affects most, if not all, of the exocrine glands of the body. The secretory functions of the sweat, salivary and pancreas glands, as well as those of the bronchioles, gastro-intestinal tract and bile-duct epithelia are known to be involved, although the basic metabolic lesion is not known.

In addition to the increased concentration of sodium chloride in sweat and nails [1], several clear cut differences between normal and CF tissues, or body fluids have recently been detected: these include a macromolecule in sweat and in serum that interferes with sodium resorption in the rat parotid gland [2, 3]; a serum factor that disrupts the beat of mammalian tracheal and oyster gill cilia [4, 5]; altered red blood cell ion transport in CF patients and their parents [6]; and non-specific changes in the carbohydrate metabolism of CF cultured fibroblasts [7]. The presence of a qualitatively 'unique' antigenic constituent in cystic fibrosis, reported by Lowe [8, 9] has not been confirmed by our group, or others [10, 11, 12, 13, 14]. However, suggestive quantitative differences in the composition of tissues or body fluids from patients with this disease, as compared to controls, has been observed immunochemically [12]. In the present report, these have been extended; an increased concentration of an antigenic factor was clearly observed in extracts of tissues from patients with CF. It was identified as C-reactive protein.

[1] Supported by research grants from the John A. Hartford Foundation and the National Cystic Fibrosis Foundation.

67

Materials and Methods

Liver, pancreas and submaxillary gland from normal individuals who died from accidental or traumatic causes, and from patients with CF were obtained as soon as possible after death, usually within 10 to 18 h. They were stored frozen at $-20°$C until needed. Samples were minced and then homogenized in a high speed blendor in phosphate-buffered saline, 0.01 M, pH 7.2, usually at 400–600 mg wet weight/ml. For immunization, whole homogenates of the normal tissues were mixed with equal parts of complete Freund's adjuvant, and injected intradermally at multiple sites into donkeys [14, 15]. Booster doses were given at intervals of one month or more, and blood samples were drawn 10 to 14 days after each injection. In *all* instances, the antisera were thoroughly absorbed with lyophilized pooled normal human plasma (60–120 mg/ml) to remove antibodies to the plasma proteins. When absorption with tissues was required, appropriate homogenates in paste-form were added to the antiserum, and stirred well. This mixture was stored 1 to 3 days at $4°$C, and then clarified by centrifugation at $102,000 \times$ g for 15 min at the same temperature.

Tissue extracts for immunodiffusion testing were prepared by homogenizing samples in buffered saline at 600 mg wet weight/ml. After storage at $4°$C overnight, the suspensions were centrifuged at $102,000 \times$ g and the supernatant fluids used for the various assays. Protein was determined by the LOWRY phenol method [16], and the extracts adjusted to equivalent protein concentrations for comparative studies (usually 30–40 mg/ml). The KRAUSE and RAUNIO [17] modification of Ouchterlony's double diffusion technic was employed, using Cordis immunodiffusion cells or templates (Cordis, Miami). Catalase assays were performed by flooding the washed and dried agar layers with 0.03% hydrogen peroxide, and observing the evolution of gas bubbles. Detection of other enzymes in the immune precipitates were carried out according to technics described by URIEL*[18] and RAUNIO [19].

Antisera to C-reactive protein (CRPA) were obtained through the courtesy of Dr. HARRISON F. WOOD, and from a commercial source (Hyland, Costa Mesa, Calif.). C-reactive protein (CRP) standards from commercial sources, as well as a sample of highly purified CRP kindly supplied by Dr. LARS-AKE NILSSON were also employed.

Samples of serum were obtained from patients who were carefully diagnosed as cystic fibrotics at the University of Miami Cystic Fibrosis Clinic. A group of in-hospital, non-CF patients of similar age group were also studied. Sera from relatives of the CF patients and from blood bank donors served as other groups of controls.

Results

Comparative analyses of extracts from normal and CF tissues, including liver, pancreas, submaxillary gland, lung, spleen, kidney, adrenal gland and heart, were performed by placing them in adjacent wells of immunodiffusion plates. It was noted that no significant differences were revealed between corresponding normal and CF samples, except in the case of liver and pancreas. By direct immunodiffusion, pooled liver extracts from patients with cystic fibrosis appeared to contain 2 antigens not detectable in similarly prepared

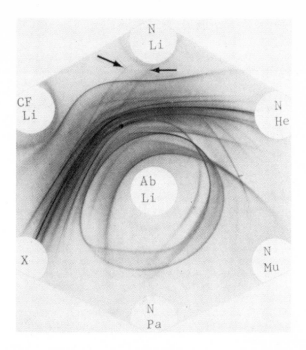

Fig. 1. Detection of 2 constituents (arrows) in the extracts of pools of livers from cystic fibrosis patients that appear to be present in higher levels than in extracts from normal, noncystic livers. N LI = normal liver; CF LI = cystic fibrosis liver; N PA = normal pancreas; N MU = normal skeletal muscle; N HE = normal heart; Ab LI = antiserum to normal liver; X = empty well.

samples from normal tissues, when tested with an antiserum to normal liver that had been thoroughly absorbed with normal human plasma (fig. 1). The same antiserum showed many more precipitin lines with CF pancreas than with the normal tissue (fig. 2). On the other hand, anti-pancreas serum revealed greater numbers of lines with normal pancreas than with the CF counterpart (fig. 3).

In order to clarify the observation noted in figure 1, the anti-liver serum was further absorbed with normal liver homogenate (400 mg wet weight/ml) until it failed to reveal any reactions with extracts of normal liver. It still showed a single crisp reaction with CF liver, as shown in figure 4. The presence in normal liver of the antigen involved is implied, since the antiserum had been developed against normal liver homogenates. The residual precipitin line was therefore

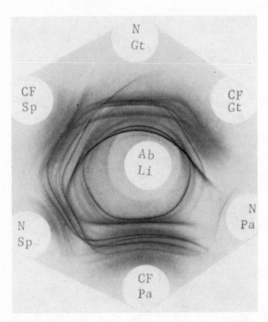

Fig. 2. Precipitin lines detected with anti-liver serum, absorbed with normal human plasma. Note the fewer numbers of lines with normal pancreas extract than with cystic fibrosis pancreas (see text). Abbreviations as before plus N Gt = normal gastro-intestinal tract; CF Gt = cystic fibrosis gastro-intestinal tract; CF Pa = cystic fibrosis pancreas; N Sp = normal spleen; CF Sp = cystic fibrosis spleen.

interpreted as being due to an antigen that is a normal constituent, but which is present in significantly higher concentrations in CF liver. For convenience it was called 'excess CF factor'.

The above studies with liver were done with pools of tissue prepared from 4 to 6 CF patients or controls. When extracts from individual livers were prepared and tested, each of the 5 CF samples showed the same reaction, while none of the 5 control livers revealed any reactivity under these conditions.

Extracts of pooled normal and CF kidneys and pancreases were also studied with such doubly-absorbed antiserum (fig. 5). Kidney and pancreas, as well as liver, from patients with this disease contained the 'excess factor', while corresponding normal tissue extracts did not.

Experiments were designed to investigate the relationship of this factor to a known 'abnormal' serum constituent, C-reactive protein (CRP). Using specific antibody, as well as purified CRP, the 'excess

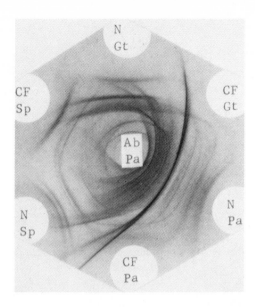

Fig. 3. Precipitin lines detected by anti-pancreas serum absorbed with normal human plasma. Note the larger number of lines with normal pancreas than with cystic fibrosis pancreas extracts (see text). Abbreviations as before.

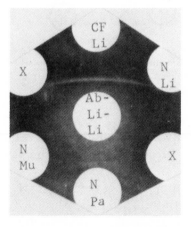

Fig. 4. Detection of the 'excess cystic factor'. Abbreviations are the same as in figure 1, except Ab-Li-Li is antiserum to normal liver absorbed with normal human plasma plus normal human liver. Note the complete absence of reaction with extracts of normal liver, and other normal tissues.

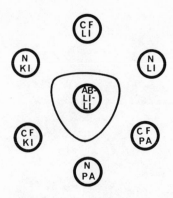

Fig. 5. Reactions between extracts of pools from cystic fibrosis liver, kidney and pancreas together with lack of reactions with the extracts from the normal counterparts, using anti-normal liver absorbed with normal human plasma plus normal human liver. Abbreviations as in figure 1 and 2 plus: N KI = normal kidney; CF KI = cystic fibrosis kidney; CF PA = cystic fibrosis pancreas.

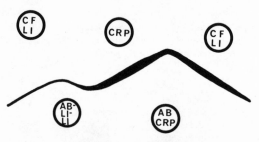

Fig. 6. 'Reactions of identity' between C-reactive protein and cystic fibrosis liver as revealed by anti-C-reactive protein and anti-normal human liver absorbed with both normal human plasma and normal human liver. Abbreviations as before, plus: CRP = C-reactive protein; Ab CRP = antiserum to C-reactive protein.

CF factor' was unequivocally identified as C-reactive protein (fig. 6). Each of the immune precipitates merged completely in 'reactions of identity'.

In view of this identification of the 'excess CF factor' as C-reactive protein, samples of sera from CF patients, their relatives and controls were studied for the presence of this protein, using known antibody to this substance. The results, summarized in table I, showed that the incidence of positive reactions was higher than had been anticipated. However, the CF patients did not reveal a greater incidence of this

Table I. Incidence of detectable C-reactive protein in the sera of various groups, as studied by two directional immunodiffusion, using anti-C-reactive protein

Group	Number Tested	Positives Number	Positives Percentage
Cystic fibrosis	45	20	44
Relatives	50	21	42
Non CF, not normal	100	59	59
Normal All	37	28	75
Normal Young	18	10	54
Normal Old	19	18	94
Normal blood bank	265	183	69

Non CF, not normal = hospitalized patients, same age distribution as the cystic fibrosis patients
normal = from persons taking their annual physical examinations and clinic check-ups
  – all = aged 3 to 55
  – young = aged 3 to 18
  – old = aged 19 to 55
normal blood bank = sera from blood bank, negative for serological tests for syphilis.

component in serum, as compared to controls and relatives. If anything, the incidence was a little lower, but age factors were not exactly equivalent among the various groups. Thus 44 % of CF patients, 42 % of relatives, 59 % of non-CF non-normal patients, and 69 % of normal (blood bank) sera contained readily detectable CRP. The latter is especially interesting in the light of the earlier concept that CRP represents an acute phase protein, present in association with tissue damage, infectious or inflammatory disease processes. The sera from the blood bank consisted of screened donors who were considered to be healthy and normal.

It has been reported that CRP is antigenically related to catalase [20, 21]. Therefore, the immunodiffusion patterns of the 'excess CF factor', such as seen in fig. 4 and 5 were tested for catalase activity. The results were quite negative.

In view of the differences in composition of normal and CF pancreas seen with these antisera (see fig. 2 and 3) and in an attempt to gain more information about the constituents of these tissues, precipitin patterns on other plates in which normal and CF tissues had been

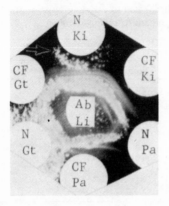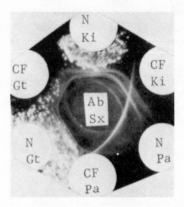

Fig. 7. Assay for catalase, using anti-liver serum. Catalase activity is indicated by bubbles of gas formed. Note 2 different areas of activity: e.g. one close to normal kidney antigen well (arrow) and a second line common to all tissues tested, except normal pancreas (see text). Abbreviations as before plus: CF Gt = Cystic fibrosis gastro-intestinal tract; N Gt = Normal gastro-intestinal tract.

Fig. 8. Assay for catalase using anti-submaxillary gland serum. Catalase activity indicated by bubbles of gas. Note activity only in the arc close to antigen wells. Abbreviations as before plus: Ab Sx = antiserum to submaxillary gland.

compared, were also tested for catalase. Whereas none of the CRP or 'excess factor' lines revealed enzymatic activity, 2 catalase zones were seen with certain tissues on plates using anti-liver serum as the antibody source (fig. 7). One of the catalase zones was present in normal, but not CF kidney (arrow), while a second catalase band was common to all the tissue extracts tested (except normal pancreas). Only the former distribution was noted in the case of these tissue extracts reacting with anti-pancreas or anti-submaxillary gland serum (fig. 8). These assays had been performed with immunodiffusion patterns using extracts of pooled tissues, but when extracts from individual normal and CF kidney were studied, catalase activity was randomly distributed among the normal and patient samples, indicating that the lack of catalase in CF kidney seen above was not related to the disease process, but appeared to be individually determined.

Other enzyme assays were performed on parallel plates comparing extracts of normal and CF tissues. One glucosaminidase and a separate glucuronidase band were detected at similar concentrations by each of the antisera in all the normal and CF tissues tested, except in the case of normal pancreas. Anti-liver and anti-submaxillary gland sera showed lines with each of these enzymatic activities in CF pancreas, but only traces of the enzymes were found in normal pancreas.

Only anti-pancreas serum revealed a cystine-amino-peptidase, and similar levels were seen in normal and CF kidney and lung. Cystic fibrosis pancreas showed patterns which indicated that this enzyme was present in lower concentrations than in the normal counterpart.

All tissues had one phosphatase system revealed by the 3 antisera, with no difference being shown between the normal and diseased tissues.

Three distinct esterases were demonstrated in most normal and CF tissues on the slides developed with anti-normal liver serum. One was detected with anti-normal submaxillary gland serum; and none was revealed by anti-pancreas serum. Of the 3 esterases seen with anti-liver serum, one was equally distributed between the normal and CF tissues. The other 2 esterases were either absent or rarely detectable in normal pancreas, but were clearly visualized in CF pancreas and the other tissues examined. Anti-submaxillary gland serum also revealed decreased levels of an esterase in normal pancreas, as compared to the CF tissue.

Discussion

The differences noted in these comparative studies of extracts of normal and CF pancreas, apparently quite striking, can be explained on a quantitative rather than qualitative basis. RAUNIO, in his studies on the composition of normal and CF pancreas by immuno-electrophoresis, also detected clear differences between the two [12]. However, reciprocal absorption studies showed that these were only quantitative, since all reactivities were abolished following these procedures. As the pancreas is usually rather atrophied in cystic fibrosis, being depleted of glandular antigens or enzymes, it would be expected to show decreased numbers of constituents with anti-pancreas serum. On the other hand, since extracts with equivalent protein concentrations were tested, proportionately greater amounts of structural proteins would be anticipated in the samples from atrophied CF pancreas, resulting in greater cross-reactivity with the non-pancreas antisera, e.g. anti-liver antiserum.

75

In the present studies, all of the extracts of cystic fibrosis liver revealed detectable C-reactive protein, while none of the controls did. However, CRP must have been present in normal liver, since the antiserum used was prepared against this tissue. The normal levels in liver had to be less that necessary for its detection in the immunodiffusion assay system used.

The source of the materials studied in the tests must also be considered. The organs from patients with cystic fibrosis were obtained at autopsy, usually after a long period of infections, tissue damage and general debilitation. Since the liver is one site of synthesis of C-reactive protein [22], it was not surprising that it could be detected in the extracts of livers from cystic fibrosis patients. By contrast, the normal liver samples were from accident victims, i.e. sudden death of apparently healthy people. It was unexpected however, that the kidney and pancreas extracts from cystic fibrosis patients would be positive for C-reactive protein. This may represent contamination of the extracts by the blood in the tissues, or storage or synthesis of C-reactive protein in these organs. However, examination of serum specimens for C-reactive protein did not reveal a higher incidence of this protein in these patients, as compared to the controls, or to their relatives, although quantitative assays of C-reactive protein were not performed. The frequent occurrence of respiratory disease in CF patients, as well as the above findings of detectable C-reactive protein levels in the tissues from this disease, suggested that the frequency of C-reactive protein detection in the serum should have been appreciably greater than the controls of similar age.

The high incidence of C-reactive protein in the older age group of normals (55% incidence in young, as compared to 90% in the older group) confirms NILSSON's observations, which showed that C-reactive protein appeared to be more frequent in normal sera with increasing age (ranging from 17% in children younger than 18 years of age to 84% of normal men aged 50) [23, 24]. The data also support those of GOTZ [25, 26] who found C-reactive protein in *all* 90 blood bank sera tested by this method. It is thus amply clear that C-reactive protein, which had long been considered an acute phase protein, synthesized only as a consequence of inflammatory or tissue damage states, actually represents a normal plasma protein, which increases in concentration significantly as a result of such disturbances. The conventional capillary tube precipitation method is much less sensitive than the immunodiffusion system used here, and had led to the assumption that C-reactive protein was not present normally. Similar considerations on the sensitivity of the methods employed may cause a re-evaluation of the composition of normal serum [27, 28]. However, these findings in no way invalidate the diagnostic usefulness of C-reactive protein determinations by the capillary tube precipitin method, since the sensitivity of this technic seems ideally suited to distinguish the elevated levels of this protein from the 'normal'. Gotz [24] reported that sera positive for C-reactive protein by the capillary tube test contained 8-10 times the concentration of this factor over that found in blood bank sera.

References

1. DI SANT'AGNESE, P. A.; DARLING, R. C.; PERERA, G. A., and SHEA, E.: Abnormal electrolyte composition of sweat in cystic fibrosis of pancreas: Clinical significance and relationship to disease. Pediatrics *12:* 549 (1953).
2. MANGOS, J. A. and McSHERRY, N. R.: Sodium transport: Inhibitory factor in the sweat of patients with cystic fibrosis. Science *158:* 135 (1967).
3. MANGOS, J. A. and McSHERRY, N. R.: Studies on the mechanism of inhibition of sodium transport in cystic fibrosis of the pancreas. Pediat. Res. *2:* 378 (1968).
4. SPOCK, A.; HEICK, H. M. C.; CRESS, H., and LOGAN, W. S.: Abnormal serum factor in patients with cystic fibrosis of the pancreas. Pediat. Res. *1:* 173 (1967).
5. BOWMANN, B. H.; LOCKHART, L. H., and McCOMBS, M. L.: Oyster ciliary inhibition by cystic fibrosis factor. Science *164:* 325 (1969).

6. BALFE, J. W.; COLE, C., and WELT, L. C.: Red cell transport defect in patients with cystic fibrosis and in their parents. Science *162:* 689 (1968).

7. DANES, B. S. and BEARN, A. G.: A genetic cell marker in cystic fibrosis of the pancreas. Lancet *i:* 1061 (1968).

8. LOWE, C. V. and NETER, E.: Chemical and serological studies on a complex carbohydrate, isolated from patients with fibrocystic disease of the pancreas. Amer. J. Dis. Child. *94:* 400 (1957).

9. LOWE, C. V.; ADLER, W.; BROBERGER, O.; WALSH, J., and NETER, E.: Mucopolysaccharide from patients with cystic fibrosis of the pancreas. Science *153:* 1124 (1966).

10. BROGLIO, A. L.; SAARI, T. N.; BLACKWELL, C.; CARLSEN, D. M., and MATTHEWS, L. W.: Comparison of stool antigens from normal and cystic fibrosis children. Presented at Cystic Fibrosis Club Conference, Atlantic City, April 26 (1967).

11. TALAMO, P. C.: Immunochemical investigations of urinary macromolecules in cystic fibrosis; in DI SANT'AGNESE Research on pathogenesis of cystic fibrosis, p. 356 (1966).

12. RAUNIO, V.: A study of soluble tissue antigens in patients with cystic fibrosis and normal controls; in DI SANT'AGNESE Research on pathogenesis of cystic fibrosis, p. 339 (1966).

13. BURGER-GIRARD, N.: Thesis, Univ. of Berne (Schwabe, Bale 1964). Etude immunologique des proteines de la salive normale et de mucoviscidose.

14. TALAMO, R. C.; RAUNIO, V.; GABRIEL, O.; PALLAVICINI, J. C.; HALBERT, S. P., and DI SANT'AGNESE, P.: Immunologic and biochemical comparison of urinary glycoproteins in patients with cystic fibrosis of the pancreas and normal controls. J. Pediat. *65:* 480 (1964).

15. HALBERT, S. P.; GREENE, E. L., and PALLAVICINI, C.: 'Tissue' antigens and enzymes in human urine. 16th Colloquium, Protides of the Biological Fluids, p. 559 (1969).

16. LOWRY, O. H.; ROSEBROUGH, N. J.; FARR, A. C., and RANDALL, R.: Protein measurement with the Folin phenol reagent. J. biol. Chem. *193:* 265 (1951).

17. KRAUSE, U. and RAUNIO, V.: Sensitivity and reproducibility of a microplate technique for immunodiffusion. Acta path. microbiol. scand. *71:* 328 (1967).

18. URIEL, J.: Color reactions for the identification of antigen-antibody precipitates in gel diffusion media; in Methods of immunology and immunochemistry. III (Academic Press, New York 1968).

19. RAUNIO, V.: Characterization of glycosidases by immunoelectrophoresis. Acta path. microbiol. scand. suppl. 195 (1968).

20. HOKAMA, Y.; CROXATTO, H. D.; YAMADA, K., and NISHIMURA, E. T.: The occurrence of immunologically common antigenic components in C-reactive protein and human hepatic and erythrocyte catalase. Cancer Res. *27:* 2300 (1967).

21. NISHIMURA, E. T.; TAKAHARA, S., and HOKAMA, Y.: Interrelationship of catalase and C-reactive protein in acatalasemic erythrocytes. Arch. Biochem. *126:* 121 (1968).

22. HURLIMANN, J.; THORBECK, G. J., and HOCHWALD, G. M.: The liver as the site of C-reactive protein formation. J. exp. Med. *123:* 365 (1966).

23. NILSSON, L. A.: C-reactive protein in apparently healthy individuals (blood donors) related to age. Acta path. microbiol. scand. *73:* 619 (1968).

24. NILSSON, L.-A. and TIBBLIN, G.: C-reactive protein in a random sample of Swedish men aged 50. Acta med. scand. *183:* 467 (1968).

25. GOTZ, H.; PEREZ-MIRANDA, M., and SCHEIFFARTH, F.: Newer findings about C-reactive protein (C-reactive protein a normal seraprotein?) 17th Colloquium, Protides of the Biological Fluids (1969).

26. GOTZ, H.; PEREZ-MIRANDA, M. und SCHIEFFARTH, F.: Antigeneigenschaften des C-reaktiven Proteins. Z. klin. Chem. u. klin. Biochem. *7:* 275 (1959).

27. GREENE, E. L.; HALBERT, S. P., and PALLAVICINI, J. C.: Studies in the origins of 'tissue' antigens and enzymes in urine (in manuscript).
28. McPHAUL, J.J., jr. and DIXON, F.J.: Immunoreactive basement membrane antigens in normal human urine and serum. J. exp. Med. *130:* 1395 (1969).

Serogroups of *Pseudomonas aeruginosa* and the Immune Response of Patients with Cystic Fibrosis

Federico Diaz, Luis L. Mosovich, and Erwin Neter

It is well known that patients with cystic fibrosis are prone to chronic infections of the respiratory tract [1, 2]. Increasingly often *Pseudomonas aeruginosa* is the responsible microorganism in both its nonmucoid and mucoid forms [2, 3]. Its contribution to the pathogenesis of the lung involvement has not been definitely ascertained [3]. It is assumed that active infection rather than surface colonization must take place in order to elicit a specific immune response. Therefore, in this study the antibody response of patients with cystic fibrosis harboring *P. aeruginosa* was determined and, in addition, all isolates were grouped serologically according to O antigens.

Subjects, Materials, and Methods

Forty patients with cystic fibrosis, ranging in age from 1 month to 20 years, were studied. All but 17 were hospitalized during the observation period of 10 months. The diagnosis was based on the history, findings on the physical examination and chest roentgenograms, abnormal concentrations of sodium in sweat, diminished or absent proteolytic

This investigation was supported by a research grant (AI-00658) from the National Institute of Allergy and Infectious Diseases, National Institutes of Health, U.S. Public Health Service.

The authors are indebted to Mrs. Thelma F. Muraschi, New York State Department of Health, Albany, New York, for providing the prototype strains of *Pseudomonas aeruginosa*. They are most grateful to their colleagues at Buffalo Children's Hospital and acknowledge with thanks the technical assistance of Mrs. Dessie McCartan, Mrs. Helga von Langendorff, and Mrs. Doris Schroeter.

activity in the duodenal juice, and abnormal vitamin A absorption tests. Three patients had meconium ileus previously, and one subject had a meconium plug. The patients received mist-tent therapy, generated by an ultrasonic nebulizer, with a 10% solution of propylene glycol, and postural drainage. Daily vitamin supplements included vitamin A (6,000 units), vitamin D (800 units), and vitamin E (50 units). Cotazym was used for pancreatic enzyme replacement therapy.

Sputum was obtained for cultural purposes bimonthly during each clinic visit and weekly during hospitalization. In 5 patients under the age of 3 years, cultures were obtained from the throat by the removal of secretions after coughing. Patients with clinical evidence of respiratory infection received therapeutic doses of antibiotics for at least 3 weeks. Oxacillin, methicillin, erythromycin, or lincomycin was used in the treatment of infection with *Staphylococcus aureus;* streptomycin, ampicillin, or chloramphenicol for the treatment of infection with *Hemophilus influenzae;* and polymyxin B, both parenterally and by aerosol, for infection due to *P. aeruginosa.* None of the strains of *P. aeruginosa* was resistant to polymyxin B. It was not the purpose of this study to evaluate this antibiotic in the treatment of cystic fibrosis or to determine whether disappearance of the pathogen from the respiratory tract was related to antibiotic therapy or occurred spontaneously.

All available patients enrolled at the Cystic Fibrosis Center of the Buffalo Children's Hospital were included in the present study.

Bacteriologic examination of sputum was carried out as follows. The specimens were seeded on blood (brain veal) agar, phenylethanol-blood agar, Endo or MacConkey agar, as well as into brain heart infusion broth. The organisms were identified by conventional methods, including tests for coagulase on staphylococci and for the characteristic pigment on *P. aeruginosa.* Repeated cultures were taken, and special attention was paid to the presence of mucoid and nonmucoid colonies of *P. aeruginosa;* all isolates of this microorganism were used to prepare O antigens for the immunological and serological studies. When mucoid as well as nonmucoid colonies were found in a given specimen, O antigens were prepared from broth. The methods for the preparation of the O antigens have been described previously [4, 5].

Serum specimens, obtained at varied intervals, were kept frozen at −20 C. Antibodies against the O antigens of *P. aeruginosa* were identified and titrated by means of the hemagglutination and hemagglutination-inhibition reactions previously described [4, 5]. Briefly, for the preparation of the O antigen, the microorganisms were grown on brain veal agar, and the growth was suspended in phosphate hemagglutination buffer. The suspension was heated in boiling water for 1 hr and then centrifuged at 23,500 g. The clear supernatant fluid, containing O antigen, was mixed with thrice-washed human red blood cells of blood group O. Under these conditions, the antigen attaches to the surface of the erythrocytes. After incubation at 37 C for 30 min, the cells were washed 3 times in phosphate hemagglutination buffer. For the titration of antibodies, serum in 2-fold serial dilutions (0.2 ml) was mixed with equal amounts of antigenically modified erythrocytes. Hemagglutination was read after incubation at 37 C for 30 min and centrifugation at 1,300 g for 2 min. The highest serum dilution yielding hemagglutination was taken as the end point, representing the titer of the corresponding antibodies. All sera from each patient were tested with all antigens made from each subject's isolates, both nonmucoid and mucoid, belonging to different serogroups. For control purposes, O antigens from 18 serogroups of shigellae, salmonellae, and enteropathogenic *E. coli* were used. The antibody response was considered to be significant either when the titer of antibodies against a given O antigen had increased at least 4-fold without a parallel change in the titers against the enterobacterial antigens or when the antibody titer against the O antigen of the infecting microorganism was at least 4-fold higher than the titers of antibodies against all unrelated O antigens. Sera were also tested with the 15 prototypes of *P. aeruginosa* in order to detect antibodies to other serogroups. The specificity of the antibody response was documented by hemagglutination-inhibition tests, as described previously [4, 5].

The serogroups of isolates of *P. aeruginosa* were determined by means of the hemagglutination test described above, with antisera prepared in this laboratory against the O antigens established by Verder and Evans [6] and by Habs [7] and as correlated by Muraschi et al. [8]. Prototype cultures were obtained through the courtesy of Mrs. T. F. Muraschi (New York State Department of Health, Albany). To facilitate serogrouping of the isolated strains, 3 pools of antisera were prepared as follows: pool A—antisera to Verder's serogroups II, III, IV, X; pool B—antisera to Verder's serogroups I (abc), I (acd), VI, VII; and pool C—antisera to Verder's serogroups V, VIII, IX and Habs' serogroups 4 and 10. The final dilution of each antiserum in the pool was 1:500. All strains were first screened with the 3 pools and then grouped with the corresponding individual antisera in dilutions of 1:500 and 1:2,500.

Results

The present investigation, conducted over a period of 10 months, is concerned with the serogroups of *P. aeruginosa* encountered in patients with cystic fibrosis and with the antibody response of these subjects. In all, 40 patients were studied. The patients ranged in age from one month to 20 years, the mean age being 9.3 years. There were 31 males and 9 females, the sex distribution remaining unexplained. The clinical status was rated as minimal or mild in 26 patients and moderate or severe in 14 subjects, according to the evaluation of Shwachman and Kulczycki [9].

P. aeruginosa was isolated from 31 (77.5%) of the 40 patients. In 7 patients, cultures for Pseudomonas, after 1–5 positive cultures, became negative during the observation period. Whether the disappearance was related to antibiotic therapy was not determined. Mucoid isolates of *P. aeruginosa* were found in 18 or 58% of the 31 infected patients. In all, 176 isolates were recovered; 109 or 62% were of the nonmucoid type, and 67 or 38% were mucoid. Further analysis showed that serogroups II, III, and IV accounted for 48 or 27.3% of the isolates, and serogroups I, VIII, IX, X, and 4 for an additional 49 (27.8%). With the method employed, 79 (44.9%) of the cultures could not be grouped. It is quite likely that utilization of other methods, particularly bacterial agglutination tests at 50 C, would have reduced the number of nongroupable strains. The distribution of the serogroups is recorded in tables 1 and 2. It may be seen from table 1 that serogroups II, III, and IV, alone or in combination, accounted for the infection in 66% of all patients with groupable strains. It is also evident that 2 or more serogroups were isolated from 6 or 28.6% of these same subjects. The data summarized in table 2 show that nongroupable strains alone were present in approximately 32% and together with groupable strains in an additional 42% of all infected subjects.

The patterns of persistence of infection with *P. aeruginosa* could be determined in 13 patients who were studied for at least 3 months (table 3). It is evident that in these patients the same serogroup persisted, either alone (pattern A) or interspersed with others (pattern B). Five patients exhibited pattern A and 8 pattern B. It is of particular interest to note that, without exception, mucoid and nonmucoid isolates recovered from a given patient belonged to the same serogroup.

Study of the antibody response against *P. aeruginosa* of the 24 available patients (7 patients being lost due to death or not available for blood specimens) revealed that a specific antibody response could be documented in 17 (70.8%) of

84

Table 1. Serogroups of *P. aeruginosa*, excluding nongroupable isolates, in 21 patients with cystic fibrosis

Serogroups			Number and % of patients		
II alone	5	23.8%			
II + IV	1	4.8%	8	38.1%	
II + others	2	9.5%			14 ··· 66.7%
III or IV alone	3	14.3%	6	28.6%	
III or IV + others	3	14.3%			
Others alone	7	33.3%			
Total	21	100.0%			
Single serogroups	15	71.4%			
Multiple serogroups ...	6	28.6%			

Table 2. Serogroups of *P. aeruginosa*, including nongroupable isolates, in 31 patients with cystic fibrosis

Serogroups	Number and % of patients	
NG* alone	10	32.3%
NG + II, III, or IV	5	16.1%
NG + others	3	9.7%
NG + II, III, IV, or others ...	5	16.1%
II, III, or IV	4	12.9%
Others	4	12.9%
Total	31	100.0%

{ NG + II, III, or IV; NG + others; NG + II, III, IV, or others } = 13 → 41.9%
{ II, III, or IV; Others } = 8 → 25.8%

* NG = nongroupable.

Table 3. Patterns of persistence of *P. aeruginosa* serogroups in patients with cystic fibrosis

Subjects	Months									
	1	2	3	4	5	6	7	8	9	10
	Serogroups									
Pattern A:										
Patient 15	III	...	III	III	...	III	III	...	...	...
Patient 7	X	...	X	...	X	X	X	...	...	X
Pattern B:										
Patient 4	NG*	...	NG	II,NG	NG	II,NG	II,NG	NG	II,NG	NG
Patient 1	IX	IX	...	...	IX	NG,IX	IX	NG,IX	II	II
Patient 26	NG,4	IV,4	IX,4	4	4	4	NG,4	...	...	...

* NG = nongroupable.

86

Table 4. Antibody responses to 6 different serogroups of *P. aeruginosa*

Serogroups	Dates of blood specimens		
	7-16-68	8-20-68	11-27-68
III	800*	800	800
IV	160	320	1,280
V	200	100	200
IX	20	80	160
4	160	320	1,280
NG	40	20	< 20

* Reciprocal titers.

the available 24 subjects; failure of antibody response occurred in only 7 or 29.2% of the patients. The antibodies were directed against a single serogroup in 10 subjects and against 2 or more in 7 others. An example of the latter response in a patient with multiple infections is shown in table 4. Persistent high titers were found against 2 serogroups, increasing titers against 3, and a significant decrease in titers against the sixth serogroup. Four of the serogroups to which antibodies were documented had been isolated from the patient. Further analysis (table 5) revealed that the frequency of antibody response was slightly higher in patients with multiple positive cultures than in those with only one isolation, the percentages being 76.4% and 57.1%, respectively.

In 9 patients without positive cultures for *P. aeruginosa*, the titers of antibodies detected with the prototype strains ranged from <10 to 1:40, levels found in other children without cystic fibrosis or clinical Pseudomonas infection. Finally, it is noteworthy that there was no major difference in the rates of isolation of *S. aureus* between groups infected or not infected with *P. aeruginosa*. *S. aureus* was present in 86% of patients with infection due to nonmucoid *P. aeruginosa*, in 94% of the subjects with mucoid isolates, and in 100% of those without *P. aeruginosa* in the respiratory tract.

Table 5. Relationship between the number of positive cultures and the frequency of antibody response

Antibody response	No. of positive cultures			
	Single		Multiple	
	No. and % of subjects			
Present	4	(57.1%)	13	(76.4%)
Absent	3	(42.9%)	4	(23.6%)
Total	7	(100.0%)	17	(100.0%)

Discussion

Patients with cystic fibrosis frequently harbor coagulase-positive staphylococci in the respiratory tract. More recently, *P. aeruginosa* is encountered with undue frequency in these patients, possibly because, in part, they are kept alive for longer periods of time than heretofore, and/or because of the chemotherapy used in these subjects. When present, neither staphylococci nor *P. aeruginosa* frequently cause purulent infection elsewhere or invasion of the blood stream. Pseudomonas bacteremia is far less common in this disease than in patients with leukemia. The question whether *P. aeruginosa* in the sputum of patients represents the result of surface (lumen) colonization or actual infection with involvement of the tissues may be answered, to some degree at least, by the study of the immune response of the patients.

In the present study, serogrouping based on identification of the O antigens was performed on all isolates. It is of considerable interest to note that serogroups II, III, and IV accounted for the infection in approximately 67% of all patients with groupable strains. This preponderance is not characteristic of infection in patients with cystic fibrosis alone. In a study now in progress, 58% of 84 strains of *P. aeruginosa* recovered from children with diseases other than cystic fibrosis belonged to the identical serogroups. Similar findings were obtained in a group of subjects with neoplastic diseases studied simultaneously in the same community [10]. In addition, previous investigations on humans, animals, and environmental materials revealed that these 3 serogroups accounted for approximately ⅓ to ½ of all strains [6, 7, 11–15]. It is also noteworthy that in the majority of patients with cystic fibrosis the identical serogroups could be isolated repeatedly over a period of several months, occasionally associated with the temporary appearance of other serogroups. In this connection it may be mentioned that previous studies [1, 16] revealed persistence of the same phage type of *S. aureus* in a given patient with cystic fibrosis.

Of particular interest is the finding that, invariably, mucoid and nonmucoid strains of Pseudomonas isolated from a given patient shared the identical O antigens. This finding suggests that mucoid strains may be variants of nonmucoid strains. Doggett and associates [17–19] have identified a particular capsular material produced by this mucoid variety in patients with cystic fibrosis. It is of considerable interest that the mucoid substance produced by strains isolated from patients with other diseases appears to be different. The precise reason why these mucoid varieties are so frequently found in patients with cystic fibrosis and only rarely in other subjects remains to be elucidated. Conceivably, metabolic conditions exist that favor this change. Our studies have revealed another observation of interest, namely, a relationship between infection with strains of mucoid Pseudomonas and the clinical severity of the basic illness (table 6). Of the 18 patients harboring mucoid strains, 12 (66.7%) had moderate or severe illness, and 4 of these patients died during the observation period. In contrast, only 2 (15.4%) of 13 patients without infection with mucoid strains had this degree of illness, and none succumbed. Conversely, of 17 patients with minimal or mild illness only 6 harbored mucoid strains; in contrast, 12 out of 14 with moderate to severe illness did so. There was no significant difference in the age of the patients of the 2 groups, the mean ages being 8.8 years for those with and 10.2 years for those without mucoid isolates. Since in a previous report [2] a similar correlation between presence of infection with mucoid Pseudomonas and severity of the illness was not shown, further studies are needed.

Study of the antibody response of patients with cystic fibrosis and infection with *P. aeruginosa* was, undertaken primarily in order to obtain information on the host-pathogen relationships and to provide suggestive evidence for the differentiation between surface or lumen colonization and infection leading to penetration of bacterial antigen through the mucous membranes of the respiratory tract. It is recognized that microbial antigens have to pass through the layers of the mucous

Table 6. Relationship between the clinical status and the presence of mucoid *P. aeruginosa*

| | Mucoid strains of *Pseudomonas aeruginosa* | |
| | Present | Absent |
Clinical status	No. and % of subjects	
Minimal or mild	6 (33.3%)	11 (84.6%)
Moderate or severe ..	12* (66.7%)	2 (15.4%)
Total	18 (100.0%)	13 (100.0%)

* Includes the 4 patients who died during follow-up.

membrane to reach cells of the phagocytic and immune systems. A specific immune response was documented in approximately 71% of these patients. The question arises whether this response may be accounted for by the increase with age in the level of antibody titers rather than by the clinical infection, since Gaines and Landy [20] have previously reported age-dependent increases in sera from healthy human subjects. The following make this assumption unlikely. (1) The antibody titers exceeded those found in sera of children of similar ages without infection with *P. aeruginosa,* studied at the same time but not reported here; (2) parallel changes in the titers of antibodies against O groups of Pseudomonas other than that of the infecting microorganism and against O antigens of enterobacteriaceae were not observed; and, more importantly, (3) increase in the titers of O-specific Pseudomonas antibodies was seen within a period of a few months (table 4). It is noteworthy that the antibody response occurred somewhat more frequently in patients with multiple isolations (76%) than in subjects with a single positive culture (57%). It is also of interest to note that in 7 out of 17 patients an antibody response could be documented against 2 or more O groups of Pseudomonas, supporting the observation that multiple infections with the species do occur in these subjects. An antibody response to Pseudomonas in patients with cystic fibrosis was reported previously [21], specific precipitins being found, by means of the double diffusion test, in one-third of the patients. The antibodies were present only in patients harboring *P. aeruginosa* in the sputum and mainly when the isolates were of the mucoid type. Future studies should be directed toward the elucidation of the immune response to the mucoid substance produced by certain strains of *P. aeruginosa,* and particular attention should be paid to both circulating and secretory antibodies of various immunoclasses.

Summary

In order to gain a better insight into the role of *Pseudomonas aeruginosa* present in the respiratory tract of patients with cystic fibrosis, a serologic and immunologic study was carried out; all of the isolates were serogrouped, and the antibody response to the microorganism was determined. Forty patients were studied; 77% harbored *P. aeruginosa,* and in about one-half of these subjects mucoid strains were recovered. Serogroups II, III, and IV predominated, being present in 66% of 21 patients. About one-third of the subjects were infected with more than one serogroup. Prolonged bacteriological observation revealed that a given serogroup tended to persist in each patient with the occasional appearance of others. Sixty-six percent of the patients with mucoid *P.*

aeruginosa, but only 15% of those with non-mucoid isolates, presented moderate or severe illness. All 4 patients who died during the observation period harbored mucoid strains. A specific antibody response was demonstrated in 17 of 24 patients (71%). In 7 of these patients an antibody response to more than one serogroup was documented.

References

1. Huang, N. N., E. L. Van Loon, and K. T. Sheng. 1961. The flora of the respiratory tract of patients with cystic fibrosis of the pancreas. J. Pediat. 59: 512–521.
2. Feigelson, J., and Y. Pecau. 1967. Surveillance bacteriologique de l'expectoration de 22 malades atteints de mucoviscidose. Arch. Franc. Pediat. 24:1135–1147.
3. Di Sant'Agnese, P. A., and R. C. Talamo. 1967. Pathogenesis and physiopathology of cystic fibrosis of the pancreas (concluded). Fibrocystic disease of the pancreas (mucoviscidosis). New Eng. J. Med. 277:1399–1408.
4. Neter, E., O. Westphal, O. Lüderitz, and E. A. Gorzynski. 1956. The bacterial hemagglutination test for the demonstration of antibodies to enterobacteriaceae. Ann. N.Y. Acad. Sci. 66:141–156.
5. Neter, E., A. M. Drislane, A. H. Harris, and G. T. Jansen. 1959. Diagnosis of clinical and subclinical salmonellosis by means of a serologic hemagglutination test. New Eng. J. Med. 261:1162–1165.
6. Verder, E., and J. Evans. 1961. A proposed antigenic schema for identification of strains of *Pseudomonas aeruginosa.* J. Infect. Dis. 109:183–193.
7. Habs, I. 1957. Untersuchungen über die O-Antigene von *Pseudomonas aeruginosa.* Z. Hyg. Infektionskr. 144:218–228.
8. Muraschi, T. F., D. M. Bolles, C. Moczuiski, and M. Lindsay. 1966. Serologic types of *Pseudomonas aeruginosa* based on heat-stable O antigens: correlation of Habs' (European) and Verder and Evans' (North American) classifications. J. Infect. Dis. 116:84–88.
9. Shwachman, H., and L. L. Kulczycki. 1958. Long-term study of one hundred five patients with cystic fibrosis. Amer. J. Dis. Child. 96:6–15.
10. Diaz, F., and E. Neter. 1969. *Pseudomonas aeruginosa:* serogroups and antibody response of patients with malignancy. Bact. Proc., p. 87.

11. Veron, M., and J. Corlet. 1961. Sur l'agglutination de *Pseudomonas aeruginosa:* subdivision des groupes antigéniques 0:2 et 0:5. Ann. Inst. Pasteur (Paris) 101:456–460.

12. Wahba, A. H. 1965. Hospital infection with *Pseudomonas pyocyanea:* an investigation by a combined pyocine and serological typing method. Brit. Med. J. 1:86–89.

13. Thörne, H., and A. Kyrkjebö. 1966. Serological group differentiation of *Pseudomonas aeruginosa* from various sources. Acta Vet. Scand. 7:289–295.

14. Matsumoto, H., T. Tazaki, and T. Kato. 1968. Serological and pyocine types of *Pseudomonas aeruginosa* from various sources. Jap. J. Microbiol. 12:111–119.

15. Sandvik, O. 1960. Serological comparison between strains of *Pseudomonas aeruginosa* from human and animal sources. Acta Path. Microbiol. Scand. 48:56–60.

16. Pittman, F. E., C. Howe, L. Goode, and P. A. Di Sant'Agnese. 1959. Phage groups and antibiotic sensitivity of *Staphylococcus aureus* associated with cystic fibrosis of the pancreas. Pediatrics 24:40-42.

17. Doggett, R. G., G. M. Harrison, and E. S. Wallis. 1964. Comparison of some properties of *Pseudomonas aeruginosa* isolated from infections in persons with and without cystic fibrosis. J. Bact. 87:427–431.

18. Doggett, R. G., G. M. Harrison, R. N. Stillwell, and E. S. Wallis. 1965. Enzymatic action on the capsular material produced by *Pseudomonas aeruginosa* of cystic fibrosis origin. J. Bact. 89:476–480.

19. Doggett, R. G., G. M. Harrison, R. N. Stillwell, and E. S. Wallis. 1966. An atypical *Pseudomonas aeruginosa* associated with cystic fibrosis of the pancreas. J. Pediat. 68:215–221.

20. Gaines, S., and M. Landy. 1955. Prevalence of antibody to Pseudomonas in normal human sera. J. Bact. 69:628–633.

21. Burns, M. W., and J. R. May. 1968. Bacterial precipitins in serum of patients with cystic fibrosis. Lancet 1:270–272.

Serum Precipitins to *Aspergillus fumigatus* in Cystic Fibrosis

Robert H. Schwartz, MD;
Douglas E. Johnstone, MD,
Douglas S. Holsclaw, MD, and
Richard R. Dooley, MD,

In 1967, Mearns et al[1] reported that 31% of 112 patients with cystic fibrosis seen in London hospitals had serum precipitins to antigenic extracts of *Aspergillus fumigatus*. This report stimulated a search for such antibodies in the serum of cystic fibrosis patients residing in the United States.

Methods

The primary *A fumigatus* isolate was obtained from a patient with cavitary tuberculosis complicated by a fungus ball (aspergilloma). The antigen was prepared according to the method of Longbottom and Pepys.[2] Three to five week cultures at 37 C in Sabouraud's glucose-peptone broth yielded an optimum antigen content. C-substance was present in the preparation as evidenced by broad C-substance/C-reactive substance bands in immunodiffusion. However, these nonspecific lines were distinctly different from the fine discrete antigen-antibody precipitin reactions. Cultures ·were Seitz-filtered, dialyzed against tap water, and lyophylized. The antigen was used in concentrations of 30 mg/ml in saline. Because of the high incidence of precipitins to extracts of *Staphylococcus, Pseudomonas,* and *Hemophilus,* in the serum of cystic fibrosis patients,[3,4] the fungus culture was monitored for these organisms. Microimmunodiffusion in 1% agar was used to detect precipitins. Unconcentrated serum filled a 12 mm well separated from a 4 mm antigen well by a distance of 6 mm. When antibody is present precipitin lines develop at 25 C in 24 to 48 hours.

Sera from 141 cystic fibrosis patients were examined (16, age 1 to 5 years; 36, age 6 to 10 years; 36, age 11 to 15 years; 38, age 16 to 20 years; 15, age 21 to 28 years). These were received from three Cystic Fibrosis Centers (Rochester, NY, Los Angeles, and Boston). Clinical status of patients was rated according to the system of Shwachman and Kulczycki.[5]

Results

In the cystic fibrosis group 43 of 141 (31%) sera had precipitating antibodies to *Aspergillus.* The incidence of positivity was similar for patients from Rochester, NY, Los Angeles, and Boston clinics (Table 1). Some sera also had precipitins to extracts of *Candida* or *Pseudomonas;* however, no reactions of identity or partial identity were observed with the *Aspergillus* precipitin system. *Aspergillus* precipitins were also found in the serum of three patients

with known *A fumigatus* infections. One was a boy with chronic granulomatous disease complicated by an *Aspergillus* brain abscess. The second was a patient with cavitary tuberculosis and an aspergilloma. A third had carcinoma of the lung as primary disease. Of 25 (age 15 to 25 years) young asthmatics, none had serum precipitins. Twenty-five normal (age 16 to 20 years) control sera were also negative.

The incidence of precipitins paralleled the severity of pulmonary disease. Sera from 13 of 16 patients with severe cystic fibrosis were positive (82%) (Table 2). Precipitins occurred in all age groups (two of 16, age 1 to 5 years; nine of 36, age 6 to 10 years; seven of 36, age 11 to 15 years; 20 of 38, age 16 to 20 years; five of 15, age 21 to 28 years).

Comment

A large proportion of cystic fibrosis patients in both England and the United States have precipitating

Table 2.—Prevalence of Precipitating Antibody vs Severity of Disease

Score*	1	2	3	4	5	Total
Total group	21	45	30	29	16	141
Antibody	3	11	7	9	13	43
%	14	24	23	31	82	31

* Score: 1 indicates excellent; 2, good; 3, mild; 4, moderate; 5, severe.

antibodies in their serum to antigens of *Aspergillus.* These antibodies are more likely to be found in patients with severe pulmonary disease. The reason for this high incidence may be the wide distribution of *Aspergillus* in nature and its ability to

Table 1.—Serum Precipitins to Fumigatus

Group	No.	Positive	Incidence %
Cystic fibrosis			
Rochester, NY	50	15	30
Boston	41	13	32
Los Angeles	50	15	30
Total	141	43	31
London[1]	112	35	31

flourish at body temperature, especially in damaged lung. Antibodies to *Aspergillus* may reflect colonization of dilated bronchioles without invasion of tissue.

Aspergillus infections occur when host ecology and resistance is altered by chronic disease such as lymphoproliferative disorders and by antibiotic or corticosteroid therapy.[6] Other host factors may determine the character of response upon exposure to the spores and antigens of this fungus. Atopic individuals may respond with bronchospasm and asthma by virtue of their predisposition to develop skin-sensitizing antibody (IgE). Those who respond with both skin-sensitizing antibody and serum precipitins may develop an entity called "allergic bronchopulmonary aspergillosis."[7] Episodes of transient pulmonary infiltrates, eosinophilia, and wheezing with low grade fever are the predominant features. Pepys[7] has postulated that an Arthus-type reaction, dependent upon antigen-antibody complexes, complement, and leukocytes can occur in lung tissue. *Aspergillus* spores, measuring 2.5μ to 3.0μ in diameter become trapped in mucus plugs in small bronchi. Arthus reactions around these plugs are then responsible for fluffy infiltrations and bronchiectasis.

Allergic aspergillosis has been described in five cases of cystic fibrosis.[8] However, whether or not Pepys' concept of tissue injury can be applied to the ongoing progressive lung destruction in cystic fibrosis remains to be studied. The possibility is intriguing. Antigen excess is necessary for the formation of soluble antigen-antibody complexes initiating the Arthus reaction. Such conditions might be met with either *Staphylococcus* and/or *Pseudomonas* contributing the responsible antigens. These are the almost ever-present organisms in sputum of such patients whereas *Aspergillus* is cultured infrequently (14 of 141 in the present study). In addition, precipitins to *Staphylococcus* (53%) and to *Pseudomonas* (33%) are found more frequently.[3,4]

This investigation was supported by a grant from the National Cystic Fibrosis Research Foundation.

References

1. Mearns M, Longbottom J, Batten J: Precipitating antibodies to *Aspergillus fumigatus* in cystic fibrosis. *Lancet* 1:538-539, 1967.

2. Longbottom JL, Pepys J: Pulmonary aspergillosis: Diagnostic and immunological significance of antigens and C-substance in *Aspergillus fumigatus. J Path Bact* 88:141-151, 1964.

3. Burns MW, May JR: Bacterial precipitins in serum of patients with cystic fibrosis. *Lancet* 1:270-272, 1968.

4. Halbert SP: Immunological aspects of cystic fibrosis. *Mod Prob Pediat* 10:144-157, 1967.

5. Shwachman H, Kulczycki LL: Long-term study of 105 patients with cystic fibrosis: Studies made over a five- to 14-year period. *Amer J Dis Child* **96:**6-15, 1958.

6. Finegold SM, Will D, Murray JF: Aspergillosis: A review and report of 12 cases. *Amer J Med* **27:**463-482, 1959.

7. Pepys J: Hypersensitivity diseases of the lungs due to fungi and organic dusts, in *Monographs in Allergy.* Basel, Switzerland, S Karger, 1969.

8. Batten JC: Allergic aspergillosis in cystic fibrosis. *Mod Prob Pediat* **10:**227-236, 1967.

Family adaptation to the child with cystic fibrosis

Audrey T. McCollum, M.S., and Lewis E. Gibson, M.D.

THE LIFE EXPECTANCY of children with cystic fibrosis has been significantly extended by increasingly effective medical management. However, danger exists that this increased life span may constitute little more than an attenuated death, with a highly destructive impact upon the family. Such a danger is evidenced by the observations of Lawler and associates,[1] as well as those of

Supported by United States Public Health Service Grant No. FR-00125-05 and grants from the Department of Health, State of Connecticut, and the National Cystic Fibrosis Research Foundation.

Spock and Stedman,[2] that children with cystic fibrosis have marked anxiety, preoccupation with death, and depressive trends. Lawler and associates[1] have also observed depression in parents of these children. Turk[3] has reported feelings of social isolation, reduction in intrafamilial communication, and disturbances of sexual relationship among parents.

A crucial responsibility of the professional caretakers of the child with cystic fibrosis, concomitant with the extension of life, is to determine how the psychological and social onus of this disease may be reduced. Systematic study is needed to determine the critical tasks of adaptation challenging patient and family, not only in relation to the vicissitudes of the disease but also in relation to the successive phases of childhood development. A study of family adaptation to cystic fibrosis in children is in progress in the Yale Cystic Fibrosis Service. Findings from the first phase of this study are reported here.

STUDY POPULATION AND METHODS

The population studied included 56 families of 65 living children with cystic fibrosis. These families included 87 siblings free of the disease (50 who were older than the firstborn fibrocystic child and 37 who were younger). Five other siblings with cystic fibrosis had died before the families were known to us. Thirty-four (61 per cent) families had no further children after the illness of the first fibrocystic child was diagnosed. Twenty-two (39 per cent) families had continued to reproduce, giving birth to 27 healthy infants and 5 with cystic fibrosis. These families, all Caucasian, had diverse socioeconomic characteristics, such as educational attainment, occupation, and income. Nine couples had been divorced or separated and one mother had been widowed; 46 families were structurally intact. Distribution of fibrocystic children by age and sex is indicated in Table I. Age at diagnosis is indicated in Table II.

Information was derived from 3 sources. A multiple-choice questionnaire concerning the characteristics and management of children with cystic fibrosis was completed by parents of 49 children. Parents of 55 children were interviewed by a psychiatric social worker (A. M.) to explore the issues

concerning the disease that were of particular significance to each family. Parents of 37 children participated in monthly group discussions conducted by the pediatrician (L. G.) and social worker; 24 meetings have been held. Information concerning each family has been available from at least 2 of these 3 sources. All quantified data to be reported have been derived from the questionnaire.

FINDINGS

The adaptation of parents to their children's disease appeared to progress through 4 major stages: prediagnostic, confrontational, long-term adaptive, and terminal. Since few study children have died while the study has been in progress, the terminal period will not be examined in this presentation.

PREDIAGNOSTIC STAGE

This stage represented the period between the time when parental concern about the child's health was first aroused and the time at which the correct diagnosis was established. The mean duration of this stage was 17½ months, the longest duration being 8 years. Symptoms arousing concern included one or (usually) several of the following: failure to thrive; voracious appetite; persistent fretfulness; abdominal pain; foul, bulky, fatty stools; persistent runny nose;

Table I. Distribution of study children by age and sex

Age	No. of boys	No. of girls	Total
0-4 yr.	12	13	25
5-9 yr.	19	9	28
10 yr. and over	5	7	12
Total	36	29	65

Table II. Distribution of study children by ages at diagnosis

Age at diagnosis	No. of children
0-1 yr.	
Neonatal period, 10*	33
First 6 mo., 11	
Second 6 mo., 12	
1-2 yr.	7
2-3 yr.	8
3-4 yr.	6
4-5 yr.	2
5-6 yr.	3
6-7 yr.	0
7-8 yr.	4
8-9 yr.	1
Over 9 yr.	1
Total	65

*Includes 5 younger siblings of children with cystic fibrosis.

"wheezing"; and cough. (Neonatal meconium ileus was singular as a symptom, since it always resulted in prompt diagnosis.) Parents repeatedly sought medical advice. Incorrect or incomplete diagnoses such as celiac disease, allergic reaction, asthma, bronchitis, or parental overconcern resulted in treatment which failed to ameliorate the symptoms. This often prolonged the prediagnostic stage and generated in parents a mounting mistrust of, and hostility toward, the medical profession.

Perhaps even more crucial, this stage exerted significant influence on the developing parent-child relationship. There was usually profound disturbance in the feeding situation, which constitutes the nucleus of the early mother-child relationship and is usually the earliest source of mutual gratification. Eighty-four per cent of undiagnosed children were characterized as having been voracious feeders who nonetheless failed to thrive during their first 3 months of life. These infants were unsatisfied by their feeds and had prolonged periods of fussiness. They were difficult to comfort. In 64 per cent of the group, these characteristics persisted through the first year. In the mothers, initial feelings of self-doubt and self-reproach at the incapacity to nurture the infant successfully led to feelings of despair and moments of frank hostility towards the infant. These feelings were reinforced when other symptoms such as foul stools or a persistent, intrusive cough were present, and guilt was intensified when the next stage was reached.

CONFRONTATIONAL STAGE

This stage, variable in duration, represented the period of acute stress associated with the confirmation of the diagnosis. The threat of a potentially fatal illness in the child stimulated in parents an acute, anticipatory mourning reaction. This appeared to parallel in some respects reactions which we have observed in parents of 50 children with other potentially fatal illnesses (nephrosis, solid tumors, leukemia, cardiac disease, and lupus erythematosus) and which others have described.[4-6]

Initially, defenses were mobilized to ward off recognition of the child's danger. The use of isolation was sometimes reflected in a transient detachment or absence of apparent affect. There were feelings of disbelief, with an attempt to invoke denial: "Perhaps this doctor is wrong as the others were." Avoidance was both observed and reported. Repression was utilized, with screening out or prompt forgetting of the physician's communications, often followed by random seeking of information from nonprofessional sources.

As conscious awareness of the child's danger was tolerated by parents, the affective components of the anticipatory mourning experience could be identified. These intense affects were usually accompanied by sleep disturbances and often by disturbances of appetite. Intense grief was stimulated by the threatened loss of the child. Guilt was expressed, related both to the genetic transmission of the disease and to the feelings of resentment which the child's symptoms had aroused in the prediagnostic stage. Anger was experienced. Physicians who had previously failed to diagnose the illness were frequently selected objects of anger. Anger was sometimes directed toward the organized church or God in whom the parents had believed, with a consequent weakening of faith. The marital partner was at times the object of anger because of his or her genetic contribution. It was rarely observed at this stage that the ill child was the object of conscious anger.

Intense anxiety in the confrontational stage had several sources. There was anxiety related to feelings of helplessness with respect to altering the outcome of the disease, the central parental function of protectiveness being threatened. There was anxiety related to the intensity of affects experienced and concern about their management in the future. Parents questioned, "Can I cope? Are my strong feelings normal? Will I have a breakdown?" There was anxiety relating to the fact that thoughts about the child's death could stimulate thoughts about the parent's own death.

The central issue of the confrontational

stage was, of course, the possible loss of the child. However, critical associated issues were concurrently presented. The issue of further reproduction assumed urgency, with the wish to plan a baby to replace the child who might die being opposed by the wish to avoid bearing more afflicted children. The reliability of contraceptive techniques and the risk associated with sexual intercourse had to be examined. The possibility that other family members were also afflicted with the disease had to be faced. The adequacy of the physical environment for the patient's needs became an issue. Location of residence in relation to a cystic fibrosis clinical center was important and sometimes influenced the wage earner's choice of employment. The child's need for a separate bedroom to house the mist tent sometimes dictated a change of residence. The resources of the family to absorb potentially catastrophic medical expenses was also a major issue. (A study currently in progress reveals that the per annum cost of care of a child with cystic fibrosis may exceed $10,000.) Finally, therapeutic techniques including the giving of medication, postural drainage, and operating the mist tent had to be mastered by the parents.

Any of these issues, themselves generating apprehension, could also become the displaced focus of the central anxiety about the child's death. The mist tent was observed to serve most consistently as such a focus. Both retrospectively and concurrently with its introduction, parents reported fantasies that the child would suffocate in the tent. They described the tent as "isolating, damp, and chilly" and imagined that the child would experience claustrophobic reactions. The reduction of visual contact with the child was frightening: "He seems to shrink away." "It's as though he disappears." "I wonder if she's still there." There was sometimes need to determine by tactile contact that the child was still alive.

LONG-TERM ADAPTATION

The central challenge confronting parents in this stage was that of maintaining a relationship with a potentially dying child which afforded some parental gratification and fulfilled the child's physical and psychological needs. This stage was characterized by a fluctuating balance between intercurrent mourning and denial of prognosis ("I have to believe that my child will be the exception"). Although many variable factors influenced the balance (loss of other key family members, the relationship to the child prior to manifestation of symptoms, the presence of healthy children, character of the marital relationship, the severity of the disease at the time of diagnosis, etc), denial as a useful defense was invariably impeded by the intrusive characteristics of the disease. The odor of cystic fibrosis, produced by stool and flatulence, was reported by 62 per cent of the study group to be a persistent problem in spite of enzyme therapy. It was perceived as permeating the household and eliciting expressions of shame and/or disgust from the patient, his siblings, their peers, and adults. Cystic fibrosis produced characteristic sounds, including both the noise of the mist-generating compressor and the intrusive cough of the child. Cystic fibrosis had visual impact deriving from the omnipresence of therapeutic equipment, as well as environmental deterioration (mildew and peeling paint) consequent to the high humidity levels. Household activity was recurrently interrupted for therapy, the average time spent each day on therapy and maintenance of equipment being 1.6 hours. (In 57 per cent of families with intact marriages, the husband was reported to administer therapy "frequently" or "usually." In 43 per cent he participated "rarely or "never.") There were intrusions into the sleep of the family. Fifty-nine per cent of study children were reported to have intermittent sleep disturbances, usually arousing the parents; 44 per cent experienced nocturnal enuresis, often associated with disturbances of sleep. Parents reported that these intrusive characteristics recurrently stimulated awareness of the child's illness and thoughts of his death.

In each successive phase of childhood

development, critical issues arose which served as foci of parental concern. During infancy, feeding, toilet training, management of the nebulization-postural drainage regimen, and the danger of respiratory infections constituted critical issues. During the first 3 months of life, 83 per cent of study infants (24 per cent of these had been diagnosed) had the voracious appetite and associated characteristics discussed in relation to the prediagnostic stage. During the first year, among the 64 per cent who continued to manifest these characteristics, 43 per cent had been diagnosed. Feeding problems were reported to persist among 57 per cent of study children beyond the first year, although there was a shift in their nature (approximately one half were viewed as eating more than parents felt appropriate and one half, as eating too little). Feeding disturbances were evidently not readily resolved by enzyme replacement.

The persistence of parental concern about food intake is indicated by the fact that although dietary permissiveness has been prescribed in this clinic for 3 years, 66 per cent of parents reported imposing dietary restrictions on their children. In their experience, permissiveness resulted in increased frequency and foulness of stools and flatulence, with adverse social consequences. These parents also acknowledged that they perceived their children as vulnerable and needed to encourage protein intake to foster growth and enhance strength.

Bowel training was a difficult issue for 70 per cent of the parents; 44 per cent reported training to have been either "difficult" or "stormy." An additional 26 per cent altered their timetable for training because of the deviant nature of the child's stools. The tendency towards frequency and/or urgency was reported to interfere with identifying a predictable rhythm of bowel function. The feelings of disgust stimulated in parents by the foul odor were undoubtedly transmitted to some children (one mother required her child to flush the toilet continuously while expelling the stool). Eighty-one per cent of parents continued visual inspection of the

child's stools well into the school years.

Difficulties in the management of postural drainage and nebulization were manifested between 6 and 30 months. Among those treated during infancy, 63 per cent were reported to respond with protest and resistance. Peak periods of protest occurred between 6 to 12 months and between 24 to 30 months. The powerful surge of development towards gross motor mastery and autonomy between 6 to 12 months, the tendency to protest bodily restraint, the fears associated with spatial orientation in unaccustomed positions, and dislike of manipulations around the face all appeared to be contributing factors in the earlier period. Between 24 and 30 months, characteristic negativism and assertiveness readily became attached to the regimen.

The danger of respiratory infection was a chronic focus of apprehension from infancy onward. It was necessary to weigh continuously the value of experiences such as shopping trips and contact with peers against the risk of exposure. When infections were introduced into the household, acute fear was aroused that the life of the child with cystic fibrosis would be jeopardized.

Major developmental requirements for children between 4 and 7 years of age include the loosening of intense attachments to the parents and the development of a capacity for independent function outside of the home. Although 47 per cent of study parents acknowledged that they had permitted their child less independence than they would have had he been healthy, only one child had a frank school avoidance problem. Forty-four per cent had adjustment problems in the first year of school which included inattentiveness, daydreaming, restlessness, and disturbing classroom behavior. It can be suggested but not concluded that heightened anxiety about bodily intactness in the fibrocystic child may have contributed to these problems.

Between 8 and 12 years, 2 critical issues have been identified. First, and apparently in association with the strong developmental thrust towards consolidation of peer relationships, study children had heightened awareness of and sensitivity about differences from their peers. This resulted in expressions of shame about the perceptible manifestations of the disease. Flatulence and stool odor were sources of embarrassment in school, as were the need to take medication and observe some dietary limitations. Spasms of coughing constituted an unwelcome focus of classroom attention. Reduced stamina afforded difficulty in competitive sports. The presence of the mist tent in the bedroom prompted uncomfortable questions from visitors. The need for the mist tent made participation in slumber parties and overnight camping appear problematical.

The second critical issue in this period concerned the child's emerging awareness of the prognosis. Apparently associated with the development in children in this age range of a concept of a personal and permanent death, highly charged questions were verbalized to the parents. Twenty-eight per cent of school-age children were reported to have asked no questions about the disease, its treatment, or prognosis. The remaining 72 per cent asked the following questions (in order of frequency): "Will I ever get over my sickness? When will I get better? What made me get sick? What is my sickness called? What is wrong in my body? Will I die from cystic fibrosis? Will I be able to marry? Will I be able to have children? Will my children have this disease?" Questions about prognosis were prompted by fund-raising appeals through the mass media or by frightening communications from classmates. As reported typically, the child, on return from school, might say, "Johnny told me today that I'm going to be dead by next year. Is that true?" Siblings on occasion made such a contribution. One younger sister, for example, was reported to terminate quarrels with the patient by proclaiming, "Never you mind, you're going to be with the angels pretty soon!" Parents able to master the grief, guilt, and anxiety stimulated by such questions characteristically responded with a statement such as, "None of us knows when

we're going to die. That's something God decides. But it's up to us to do everything possible to live as long we can, and that's why you must sleep in your tent, etc."

Approximately one third of the parents of school-age children avoided giving any information to the child about his illness. These parents recounted their fear that any communication with their child about his disease would result in direct questions about his possible death with which they would be unable to deal.

During the teen years, deviance and isolation from peers were intensified by retardation of growth and sexual development. Age-appropriate strivings for independence were thwarted by realistic dependence upon adults for medical care. The capacity of parents to support their teen-agers in seeking gratification through independent social, intellectual, or physical activities was highly variable. Four teen-agers were permitted (or encouraged) to avoid school frequently in spite of medical support of their attendance.

Compliance with the full therapeutic regimen was no longer sustained. Parents manifested a ready acquiescence to the protests of the adolescent against therapy. Although this acquiescence was rationalized in a variety of ways, underlying feelings of hopelessness about the prognosis appeared to constitute the major determinant.

DISCUSSION

Families of children with cystic fibrosis are challenged to cope with complex issues at each stage of the child's development and to manage the sadness, apprehension, guilt, and ambivalence appropriately aroused. Medical management, group discussions, and individual interviews have been found to make distinct contributions to mastery of these challenges.

Many issues of management can be resolved only between physician and parent with reference to the particular child's medical status. For example, judgement concerning the value of a peer group experience, such as nursery school attendance, compared to heightened exposure to respiratory infections, is one such issue. Sleep disturbance may reflect individual variables such as gastrointestinal discomfort, respiratory distress, inadequate management of the therapeutic regimen, or anxiety. Questions arise about the level of physical exertion which the child can be expected to tolerate and associated risks of exhaustion or salt depletion. Comprehensive medical management can reduce the intrusive characteristics of the disease. For example, although the sequelae of excessive fat intake may not be physiologically ominous after infancy, time invested in regulating enzyme therapy and diet to reduce foulness and frequency of stools, as well as flatulence, pays dividends in psychic and social well-being.

Group discussions make available to individual parents a corporate body of experience relevant to many children. Monthly sessions in this center are attended by a self-selected group. Topics for discussion are spontaneously introduced by members during the meetings. Although the professional knowledge of physician and social worker is made available when appropriate, the emphasis is upon fostering interchanges among members. Discussion of issues such as management of postural drainage with a negativistic infant, interpretation of the disease to siblings, and dealing with the anxieties of relatives reveal a variety of available solutions. Discussion of shared attitudes and feelings aroused by the disease reduces feelings of isolation experienced by individual parents. However, limitations are maintained on the depth to which the anxieties of any member of the group are explored, since exposure of the deep fears of one member can readily threaten the defenses of others.

In individual interviews with a social worker, parents are afforded an opportunity to examine their attitudes toward the afflicted child (as well as other intrafamilial relationships) in greater depth than is appropriate in the educational-supportive group process. Problems of social adaptation of the child with cystic fibrosis can be explored, and referral to appropriate resources in the home community can be effected. All 3 modes of supportive intervention offer professional persons continuous opportunity to deepen their own insights concerning the impact of cystic fibrosis upon the family.

SUMMARY

The adaptation of 56 families to 65 living children with cystic fibrosis has been explored. Methods included survey by detailed questionnaire, individual parent interviews, and monthly group discussions. Family adaptation progressed through prediagnostic, confrontational, long-term adaptive, and terminal stages. The first 3 have been described (the fourth is under continuing study).

The prediagnostic stage was marked by a typically prolonged period of parental anxiety before the diagnosis was established and was attended by characteristic disturbances in the feeding situation. In the confrontational stage an acute, anticipatory mourning reaction was experienced. The critical issues presented aroused a variety of intense affective responses. In the stage of long-term adaptation, denial as a useful defense was impeded by the intrusive characteristics of the disease. The management of the child with cystic fibrosis was attended by critical issues associated with each successive phase of childhood development.

The authors wish to express appreciation to Ethelyn H. Klatskin, Ph.D., Assistant Professor of Psychology, and A. Herbert Schwartz, M.D., Assistant Professor of Pediatrics and Psychiatry, who reviewed the questionnaire for appropriateness of both structure and content.

REFERENCES

1. Lawler, R. H., Nakielny, W., and Wright, N. A.: Psychological implications of cystic fibrosis, Canad. Med. Ass. J. 94: 1034, 1966.
2. Spock, A., and Stedman, D. J.: Psychological characteristics of children with cystic fibrosis, North Carolina Med. J. 27: 426, 1966.
3. Turk, J.: Impact of cystic fibrosis on family functioning, Pediatrics 34: 67, 1964.
4. Friedman, S. B., Chodoff, P., Mason, J. W.,

and Hamburg, D. A.: Behavioral observations on parents anticipating the death of a child, Pediatrics **32**: 610, 1963.

5. Bozeman, M. F., Orback, C. E., and Sutherland, A. M.: Psychological impact of cancer and its treatment. III. The adaptation of mothers to the threatened loss of their children through leukemia. Part I, Cancer **8**: 1, 1955.

6. Solnit, A. J., and Green, M.: Psychological considerations in the management of deaths on pediatric hospital services. I. The doctor and the child's family, Pediatrics **24**: 106, 1959.

Diagnosis

Screening for Cystic Fibrosis by Testing Meconium for Albumin

A. R. R. CAIN, A. M. DEALL, and T. C. NOBLE

The importance of early diagnosis of cystic fibrosis (CF) has been stressed by many authors (e.g. Lawson, Westcombe, and Saggers, 1969; George and Norman, 1971).

Methods involved have been to test either the sweat or saliva of the infant for increased levels of sodium but neither test has proved reliable, easy, or cheap in the neonatal period.

Schutt and Isles (1968) found excessive albumin in the meconium of 9 cases of meconium ileus (due to CF) and wondered if meconium testing for albumin would be a practical screening test.

Wiser and Beier (1964) had previously found that 3 out of 5 newborn sibs of known cases of CF had increased amounts of albumin in their meconium and that all the neonates with raised levels of albumin were subsequently proved to be further cases of CF.

We are in the process of conducting a newborn screening programme to detect the presence of albumin in meconium, and we are writing this preliminary communication because one case of CF has been found in the first year of the trial.

The maternity units involved in the survey have a combined delivery rate of about 5000 babies a year.

Method

The first specimen of meconium is saved in its nappy. A smear is made of this meconium on to a glass microscope slide and thoroughly mixed with a few drops of distilled water with half an orange stick. A Labstix strip (Ames) is then placed so that the edge of each of the test areas is in the resulting mixture; the strip being held horizontally with the test areas perpendicular to the slide. The presence or absence of albumin and blood is noted, traces of either being ignored. Any baby whose meconium shows the presence of both albumin and blood has a further sample of meconium or stool tested at a later date. Any baby whose meconium contains more than a trace of albumin has further specimens of meconium and stool tested and those who are persistently positive have further investigations for CF. The time taken to perform the test is 10 to 15 seconds: it is not necessary to wait for the recommended 30 seconds to look for blood if the test is negative for albumin.

Case Report

A.M. was a forceps delivery at 37 weeks' gestation, his mother being an 18-year-old primigravida. There was no history of consanguinity. His weight was 2·51 kg, length 45 cm, head circumference 32 cm and the Apgar score at 1 minute was 9. A specimen of meconium was obtained at the age of 6 hours and showed albumin $+++$ to be present. A further specimen was obtained at 22 hours with an identical result. After this his stool changed from meconium to a normal yellow colour, though it was noted to be somewhat bulky, but all subsequent tests confirmed the presence of albumin in amounts from $++$ to $+++$. Further investigations showed no tryptic activity to be present in the stool, a sweat sodium of 95 mEq/l., and a 5-day faecal fat excretion of 6·9 g per day when being fed on a half-cream milk. A chest x-ray showed no abnormality.

At the age of 3 weeks he has started on pancreatic extracts in each feed and postural drainage with gentle percussion given before feeds. Four days later it was noted that he was beginning to cough and a few medium rales were noted at the right base. A throat swab grew a coagulase positive staphylococcus. Cloxacillin was given in addition to the physiotherapy and pancreatic extracts.

He was able to go home at the age of 4 weeks weighing 2·53 kg, his parents having previously been interviewed on a number of occasions and shown how to carry out the treatment at home. His subsequent progress has been good.

He was last seen at the age of 6 months when he weighed 6·1 kg and his chest was clear to auscultation. His chest x-ray showed no abnormality. He tended to cough with his postural drainage and when he cried. His stools were occasionally greasy and foul smelling.

His treatment consisted of pancreatic powder (Pancrex V 125 mg) with each feed, flucloxacillin suspension 62·5 mg b.d., vitamins A and D 10 drops daily, ferrous sulphate 50 mg daily, vitamin C 50 mg daily, together with regular postural drainage.

109

Discussion

The trial has now been in progress for 16 months at one hospital and for 13 months at the other, during which time there have been about 6200 births. We have detected one case of cystic fibrosis by screening but there have also been two cases of meconium ileus one of which has survived and been shown to have a high sweat sodium level. We have circulated the paediatricians in the region about the trial so that we will be notified of any children who are found to have CF who were born in either of the hospitals since the beginning of the trial. In this way we hope to find out how many cases of CF have been missed by the test. As far as we know this is the first attempt at a prospective screening programme for CF using this technique.

The time taken for the test is 10 to 15 seconds and the cost of materials is just under 2p per test. In one of the hospitals the paediatric Senior House Officer does the tests while in the other the midwives and paediatric nursing staff do them.

We hope that this limited trial will stimulate other maternity units to carry out similar surveys so that the efficiency of the method can be more rapidly assessed.

It is of interest that if we had started the trial four weeks earlier we would also have detected a case of intestinal lymphangiectasia which presented at the age of 3 weeks with gross oedema and a protein-losing enteropathy.

We would like to thank all those people who are co-operating in this survey, and, in particular Mr. C. Allister for biochemical help.

REFERENCES

George, L., and Norman, A. P. (1971). Life tables for cystic fibrosis. *Archives of Disease in Childhood*, **46**, 139.

Lawson, D., Westcombe, P., and Saggers, B. (1969). Pilot trial of an infant screening programme for cystic fibrosis: measurement of parotid salivary sodium at 4 months. *Archives of Disease in Childhood*, **44**, 715.

Schutt, W. H., and Isles, T. E. (1968). Protein in meconium from meconium ileus. *Archives of Disease in Childhood*, **43**, 178.

Wiser, W. C., and Beier, F. R. (1964). Albumin in the meconium of infants with cystic fibrosis: a preliminary report. *Pediatrics*, **33**, 115.

PULMONARY MECHANICS IN ASTHMA AND CYSTIC FIBROSIS

Alois Zapletal, M.D., Etsuro K. Motoyama, M.D., Lewis E. Gibson, M.D., and Arend Bouhuys, M.D

Aɪʀᴡᴀʏ obstruction is one of the main features of bronchial asthma and of lung disease in cystic fibrosis. Its accurate assessment is therefore important for clinical diagnosis and management. In this paper we compare the results of standard spirometric tests with those of other mechanical measurements, including maximum expiratory flow-volume (MEFV) curves

and airway conductance. Our main goal was to determine which one of these tests might be sensitive as well as practicable for the quantitation of airway obstruction in asthma and cystic fibrosis. Similar data from healthy children studied in our laboratory[1] served as reference material.

SUBJECTS AND METHODS

The patients with cystic fibrosis (16 boys, 12 girls, 7 to 18 years old) were under the care of the Cystic Fibrosis Clinic at Yale-New Haven Hospital. The diagnosis was established by clinical criteria, sweat tests, and roentgenographic patterns. The selection criteria were (1) absence of acute illness and (2) a sufficient degree of cooperation in the tests. The clinical severity of the disease was classified by one of us (L.G.) prior to the present studies, according to the criteria of Shwachman and Kulczycki.[2] The patients with bronchial asthma (12 boys, 5 girls, 7 to 14 years old) had previously been seen in the pediatric clinic but were symptom-free, or nearly so, at the time of study.

The methods were the same as those described previously.[1,3] An air-conditioned

---

Abbreviations

Cdyn: dynamic compliance
FEV: forced expiratory volume
FRC: functional residual capacity
Gaw: airway conductance
MEFV: maximum expiratory flow volume
PEFR: peak expiratory flow rate
RV: residual volume
TGV: thoracic gas volume
TLC: total lung capacity
VC: vital capacity
V̇max: maximum expiratory flow rates

Presented, in part, at the meeting of the American Thoracic Society, Houston, Texas, May 20–22, 1968.
Supported, in part, by grants from National Air Pollution Control Administration, Environmental Health Service, U.S. Public Health Service (AP-00463); National Institutes of Health (HD-00989, HD-03119); Connecticut Heart Association: Connecticut Health Department; and National Cystic Fibrosis Research Foundation.

111

volume displacement body plethysmograph*
was used for the measurement of total lung
capacity (TLC), airway conductance (Gaw),
and MEFV curves. Lung volume changes
were measured with a Krogh spirometer*
connected to the body plethysmograph.
Airflow rate at the mouth was sensed with
a heated pneumotachograph (Fleisch No. 4).
Mouth pressure was measured at a lateral
pressure tap near the mouthpiece.

Lung volumes (TLC, FRC and RV) were
derived from the plethysmograph volume
record and from measurements of TGV.
VC was read from the body plethysmograph
volume record. The highest value was used
as the result. TGV was measured 5 to 10
times at different lung volume levels. For
TLC, the average of all technically adequate
measurements was used as the result. RV
was calculated as TLC–VC; FRC was determined by direct measurement (end-expira-
tory TGV) or by adding the expiratory reserve volume to RV.

MEFV curves were obtained by recording
expiratory flow rates versus plethysmographic lung volume changes on a storage
oscilloscope. The patients inspired maximally from RV and performed a complete
and maximally rapid expiration to RV. At
least three technically satisfactory curves
were obtained, with reproducible flow rates
on the effort-independent portion of the
curve.[1] The evaluation of the curves is discussed in the section on results.

Airway conductance (Gaw) was measured
during panting[4] immediately after releasing
the shutter which was closed for the TGV
determination. Several measurements were
made at different lung volume levels in each
subject. After correction for resistance of
the breathing circuit at the mouth, Gaw
was plotted versus thoracic gas volume. Airway conductance at a lung volume equal to
FRC was read from these graphs.

In most of the patients measurements of
MEFV curves and Gaw were repeated 20
minutes after inhalation of isoproterenol
(Mistometer). Apart from the plethysmo-

---

* J. H. Emerson Co., Cambridge, Mass.

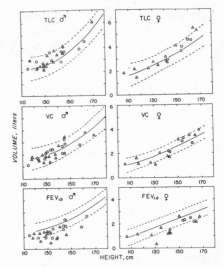

FIG. 1. TLC, VC, and $FEV_{1.0}$ in boys and girls.
Drawn and dashed lines are mean normal values ±
2 SE.[1] Triangles: patients with cystic fibrosis. Circles: patients with bronchial asthma. Same symbols
used for patients in subsequent figures.

graphic studies, we measured forced expiratory volume ($FEV_{1.0}$) with a timed spirometer, and FRC with a 7-minute helium
dilution method, using a closed circuit spirometer. TLC (helium) was calculated
from FRC by adding the inspiratory capacity (TLC_{He}). Not all measurements could

TABLE I

RV/TLC AND FRC/TLC RATIOS IN HEALTHY
CHILDREN[1] AND IN CHILDREN WITH ASTHMA
OR CYSTIC FIBROSIS

	RV/TLC	FRC/TLC
Asthma	0.28 ±0.08 (15)	0.52 ±0.04 (15)
Cystic fibrosis	0.34* ±0.13 (27)	0.54* ±0.09 (27)
Healthy ♂	0.22 ±0.061 (37)	0.47 ±0.042 (37)
♀	0.24 ±0.053 (24)	0.47 ±0.057 (24)

Data are mean ±SD. Number of subjects in parenthe-
sis.

* Significantly different from data in healthy children
(p<0.01; unpaired "t" test).

112

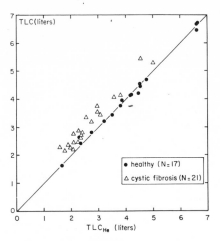

FIG. 2. TLC determined with plethysmograph (ordinate) and with gas dilution (abscissa) in normal children and those with cystic fibrosis.

be performed in all patients. This is reflected in variation of the number of subjects in different graphs.

RESULTS

Lung volumes and FEV$_{1.0}$

TLC and VC were within normal limits (i.e., the 95% confidence limits of data in healthy children) in most of our patients. FEV$_{1.0}$ was systematically lower than in comparable healthy children, and was out-

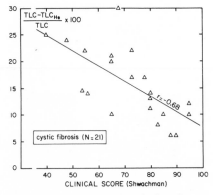

FIG. 3. Percentage gas trapping (ordinate) versus clinical score[2] (abscissa) in children with cystic fibrosis. The correlation is significant at the 1% level

side the normal limits in 10/26 patients with cystic fibrosis, and in 5/17 patients with asthma.

In asthma as well as in cystic fibrosis, TLC tended to be higher than the normal average, and VC was often near the lower limits of normal (Fig. 1). As a result, the RV/TLC ratio was often increased, as was the FRC/TLC ratio (Table I).

It is well known that air "trapping" occurs in bronchial asthma.[5] We found that it also occurs in cystic fibrosis. In these patients, TLC as measured with the plethysmograph was systematically and significantly (p < 0.001) higher than TLC$_{He}$ (Fig. 2), while the two values were nearly identical in healthy children. The difference between TLC and TLC$_{He}$ represents an amount of "trapped gas" in very poorly ventilated areas of the lungs. The amount of trapped gas correlates negatively ($r = 0.68$, p < 0.01) with the clinical condition (Fig. 3); that is, patients in poorer clinical condition tend to have more gas trapping.

Airway Conductance

Gaw at FRC (Fig. 4) was within normal limits in all patients with an FRC less than 1.5 liter. In many older children, with a larger FRC, it was abnormally low. This was true for children with asthma as well as those with cystic fibrosis.

Maximum Expiratory Flow-Volume (MEFV) Curves

These curves relate instantaneous maximum expiratory flow rates ($\dot{V}$max) at the mouth (ordinate) to lung volumes (abscissa) (Fig. 5). They are obtained during forced expirations starting from total lung capacity (right-hand side of each graph). Expiratory flow rate first rises to a peak value (peak expiratory flow rate (PEFR)) and then decreases to zero as lung volume approaches residual volume (left-hand side of each graph). Flow rates on the descending limb of the curve are independent of effort to the extent that no higher rates of flow can be achieved by increasing muscular effort during expiration.

The difference between the shape of

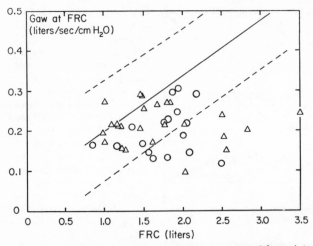

FIG. 4. Airway conductance at FRC (ordinate) versus FRC (abscissa) in children of both sexes with cystic fibrosis and with asthma. Drawn and dashed lines: mean normal values ± 2 SE.[1]

MEFV curves in healthy children and in patients of similar stature and age but with asthma or cystic fibrosis is obvious. In the examples shown, the descending limb of the curve is nearly straight in the healthy children. In many other healthy children the curve is concave toward the volume axis.[1] In contrast, this portion of the curve is convex toward the volume axis in patients with cystic fibrosis as well as in those with bronchial asthma. These patterns are representative for those observed in most of our patients. Visual inspection of the curves suggested that the decrease of flow rates at low lung volumes is often more abrupt in cystic fibrosis than in asthma. However, measurements of flow rates at different lung volumes did not show systematic and significant differences between flow rates at different points of MEFV curves in the two diseases.

Figure 6 illustrates our quantitative assessment of the MEFV curves. Figures 7 and 8 summarize its principal result. Peak expiratory flow rates were within normal limits for most patients (Fig. 7, A), but maximum flow rates at a small lung volume (25% VC) were abnormally low in 16 out of 27 boys with asthma or cystic fibrosis (Fig. 8,

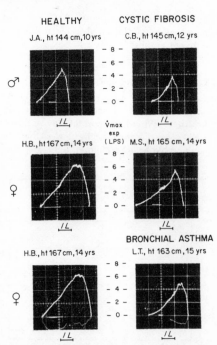

FIG. 5. Representative examples of MEFV curves in patients with cystic fibrosis or asthma, each compared with the curve of a healthy child of the same sex and similar height and age.

114

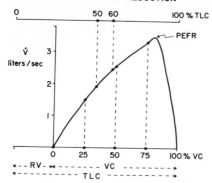

FIG. 6. Schematic MEFV curve, to show lung volume levels at which flow rates were read. TLC scale at top; VC scale at bottom.

A). At intermediate lung volumes (Fig. 6) the results were between those of Figures 7, A and 8, A. Figures 7, B and 8, B show the

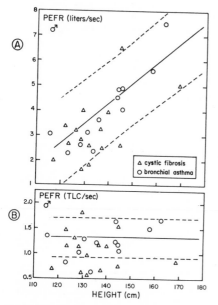

FIG. 7. A. Peak expiratory flow rate (PEFR) in male patients. Drawn and dashed lines: mean normal values ± SE[1]. B. Same data as in A, expressed in flow units of TLC/sec (see text).

same data, corrected for lung size by expressing the flow rates in units of TLC/sec instead of in liters/sec. Since TLC was larger than the average normal value in many patients, this method of plotting the data increases the number of abnormal results. The decrease of maximum flow rates is related to the clinical condition of patients with cystic fibrosis. Figure 9 demonstrates this for $\dot{V}$max at 50% TLC. In this graph, the use of flow rate units in TLC/sec eliminates the effect of lung size that otherwise makes such a relation difficult to discern.

Static Lung Recoil Pressure

This was measured, using the esophageal balloon method,[6] in a separate group of seven patients with cystic fibrosis. Satisfactory pressure-volume curves were obtained in five of these (11 to 19 years of age). Their maximum transpulmonary pressures (at full inspiration) ranged from 25 to 49 cmH₂O, which is similar to our values in healthy children and adolescents.[1] At lower lung volumes, too, these patients had static recoil pressures close to those in healthy children.

Inhalation of Isoproterenol

It is well known that bronchodilator drugs usually decrease airway obstruction in bronchial asthma. Figure 10 shows increases in flow rates on MEFV curves with isoproterenol. Twelve of 14 patients with a history of asthma showed an improvement in flow rates. In cystic fibrosis, the effect of the drug was usually minimal. It caused flow rate increases (Fig. 11, subject M.S.) in 6 of 20 patients, while in two other patients flow rates decreased after isoproterenol (Fig. 11, subject J.S.). In the latter example, $\dot{V}$max after isoproterenol decreased abruptly at a lung volume of about 50% VC.

The patients with asthma and with cystic fibrosis also differed in regard to the effect of the dilator drug on airway conductance. In 14 children with asthma, the Gaw/TGV ratio increased by 38% on the average (p < 0.01). On the other hand, in 18 patients with cystic fibrosis this ratio did not change significantly (average increase: 4%).

115

Aerosol Therapy

Seven boys and seven girls with cystic fibrosis were treated in a tent with a mist of 10% propylene glycol in distilled water during periods varying from 2 to 7 months. These patients slept in a tent 7 nights per week. Lung function tests were done at the beginning and end of the therapy period in all children. Only one patient had a clearly improved lung function at the end of therapy ($2\frac{1}{2}$ mo). Her VC increased 27%, $FEV_{1.0}$: +37% and $\dot{V}$max at 50% VC: +50%. However, in the group as a whole, no systematic improvement occurred. At low lung volumes, flow rates on MEFV curves decreased in most patients ($\dot{V}$max at 25% VC: −20%); at higher volumes they did not change systematically (e.g., $\dot{V}$max at 75% VC: −2%).

DISCUSSION

We studied a group of patients with asthma and with cystic fibrosis who were in a good clinical condition. We purposely selected such a group since we wanted to study certain indices of lung mechanics which might detect the pathological condition of the lungs in these patients at a stage where conventional tests yield results close to normal limits.

The measurement of maximum expiratory flow rates at different, in particular at small, lung volumes appears to provide such a sensitive test. Visual inspection of the MEFV curves (Fig. 5) often detects the abnormality, since their shape differs markedly from that in healthy children. MEFV curves which are convex to the volume axis are rare among healthy children. Among 65 healthy subjects, only six boys (9%) had such a curve[1] and we suspect that in them we dealt with an early effect of cigarette smoking. In the present studies nearly all patients had this convex-to-volume-axis type of curve.

Quantitative evaluation of MEFV curves, in terms of maximum flow rates at defined lung volume levels (Fig. 6), yields additional information. In healthy children, these flow rates increase in proportion to TLC over the age range 6 to 18 years: the ratio $\dot{V}$max/TLC (with $\dot{V}$max measured at any lung volume in

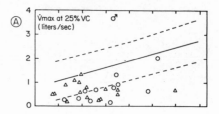
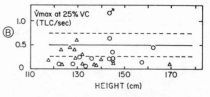

Fig. 8. A and B. Similar to Figure 7 for maximum expiratory flow rate at 25% VC.

the vital capacity range) is independent of height.[1] The rationale for the use of $\dot{V}$max/TLC ratios is that it expresses flow rates in units which are related to lung size. Our previous studies in healthy children suggest that the mechanical conditions for air flow through the airways are similar when the rates of flow constitute a certain fraction of TLC. For instance, a flow rate of 1 liter/sec through airways of lungs with a TLC of 2

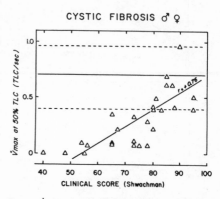

CYSTIC FIBROSIS ♂ ♀

Fig. 9. $\dot{V}$max at 50% TLC (ordinate), in TLC/sec, versus clinical score[2] (abscissa) in children of both sexes with cystic fibrosis. The correlation is significant at the 1% level.

116

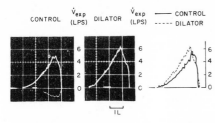

CONTROL $\dot{V}_{exp}$ (LPS)   DILATOR $\dot{V}_{exp}$ (LPS)   —— CONTROL   ----- DILATOR

FIG. 10. Improvement of maximum expiratory flow rates on MEFV curves after inhalation of isoproterenol in a symptom-free patient with bronchial asthma.

liters appears to be mechanically equivalent to a flow rate of 4 liters/sec in lungs with a TLC of 8 liters, if both flows occur at lung volumes which are comparable as a percentage of VC or TLC.

Since TLC tended to be slightly, although insignificantly, larger than normal in our groups of patients, the ratios $\dot{V}max$/TLC were more often abnormally low than was the absolute value of $\dot{V}max$ (in liters/second). For practical purposes it may be more important that the use of $\dot{V}max$/TLC ratios allows an assessment of pulmonary function which is independent of height. If one obtains both MEFV curves and TLC at intervals during prolonged periods of observation, changes in the degree of airway obstruction may be assessed, even though growth of the patient alters the absolute values of $\dot{V}max$ and TLC.

The decrease of maximum expiratory flow rates in our patients was pronounced at low lung volumes (compare Figures 7 and 8). If we consider the test with the highest incidence of abnormal results as the most sensitive index of disease, $\dot{V}max$ at 25% VC is clearly the most sensitive test in our study. It gave 58% abnormally low values among all patients, compared with 41% for RV/TLC, 35% for $FEV_{1.0}$ and 10% for PEFR.

DeMuth et al.[7] found abnormal N_2 washout curves in children with cystic fibrosis who had no clinical evidence of lung disease, and whose VC, RV, and maximum breathing capacity were within normal limits. Such results suggest uneven distribution of ventilation resulting from nonuniform degrees of obstruction of small airways. This type of obstruction can also account for our findings. Obstruction of peripheral airways decreases maximum expiratory flow rates, while airway conductance may show only a slight decrease or may not decrease at all.[8,9] This is because the total cross-section area of peripheral airways is very large. Airway conductance is thus determined chiefly by large airways with a smaller aggregate cross-section area. Maximum flow rates, on the other hand, decrease when small airways are obstructed since the supply of air from terminal lung units is a main determinant of maximum flow.

Another explanation of the decreased maximum flows might be loss of lung elastic recoil. Elastic recoil pressure is an important component of the driving pressure for maximum flow[10,11] and its decrease probably accounts, in part, for the low maximum flow rates in emphysema. Our data are not sufficient to reject this mechanism in the case of cystic fibrosis. However, at least a few patients had low flow rates and normal static lung recoil pressures. In addition, pathological studies have shown little or no evidence of destructive emphysema in lungs from patients with cystic fibrosis.[12] Loss of elastic recoil, therefore, is probably unimportant as a cause of low maximum flow rates in most patients with cystic fibrosis. In asthma the ready reversibility of diminished expiratory flow rates by β-stimulant drugs such as isoproterenol suggests that small airway obstruction by bronchospasm is the major cause of low flow rates on MEFV curves in that disease.

Yet another mechanism which may lead to decreased maximum expiratory flow rates involves changes of the compliance of large airways. It has been suggested[13] that large airway collapse is common in cystic fibrosis]. However, such a collapse is a normal accompaniment of forced expirations.[9] There is at present no convincing evidence that the compliance of large airways differs in health, in asthma, and in cystic fibrosis. It is possible, though, that the decrease of $\dot{V}max$ after a bronchodilator drug in two patients (Fig. 11, J.S.) is related to an increase of large airway

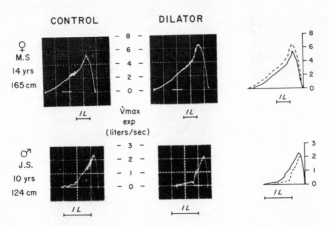

CONTROL   DILATOR

♀
M.S
14 yrs
165 cm

Vmax
exp
(liters/sec)

♂
J.S.
10 yrs
124 cm

FIG. 11. Effect of isoproterenol inhalation in two patients with cystic fibrosis. Slight improvement of flow rates on the MEFV curve resulted in subject M.S. In contrast, flow rates decreased after this drug in subject J.S.

compliance by this drug. Relaxation of smooth muscle may render large airways more compressible and this may decrease $\dot{V}$max.[14] The lack of change of $\dot{V}$max and of Gaw after isoproterenol in most patients with cystic fibrosis suggests that the structural damage to the airway wall and/or presence of mucous secretions in the airways are more important determinants of lung mechanics than alterations of its smooth muscle tone. Our data do not support the general use of bronchodilator drugs in patients with cystic fibrosis, as recommended by others.[15]

We have been unable to demonstrate objective functional improvement in some of our patients after aerosol therapy in a mist tent. These results are in agreement with the findings in a separate group of 16 children with cystic fibrosis in whom serial studies of MEFV curves and $FEV_{1.0}$ were performed during the periods when their therapy did or did not include mist therapy.[16] In these studies there was a tendency toward improvement when the patients were not receiving mist tent treatments. The positive results obtained with mist therapy reported by others[17] were in part based on changes in

FRC/TLC ratio where TLC was measured with helium dilution. The present study demonstrated that in patients with lower airway obstruction FRC measurements with the helium dilution method gave erroneously low values due to air trapping (Fig. 2). The FRC/TLC ratio is therefore not reliable unless volumes are measured with a body plethysmograph.

Mellins, et al.[13] have suggested that airway obstruction is less uniform and involves larger airways in cystic fibrosis than in asthma. Our data do not permit such a conclusion. We have been unable to detect systematic differences in pulmonary mechanics between patients with the two diseases. In both, flow rates at low lung volumes are predominantly decreased.

SPECULATION

We must consider the possibility that part of the functional abnormality in our patients may be related to development arrest caused by the disease process.[18] It may be of interest that the younger children had normal conductance values; the data of Figure 4 could be interpreted as showing lack of increase of conductance during growth in the patients.

Further evidence on this point should be sought, perhaps through prospective studies.

SUMMARY

We believe that MEFV curves offer a simple and sensitive quantitative assessment of small airway obstruction in bronchial asthma and cystic fibrosis. Previous studies have shown their value in the detection of minor degrees of airway obstruction induced by broncho-constrictor agents.[8,19] Woolcock, et al.[20] have suggested that small airway obstruction may manifest itself principally in frequency-dependence of dynamic compliance [$Cdyn^1$]. However, their own data show good correlation between frequency-dependence of $Cdyn^1$ and maximum mid-expiratory flow. It is well known that N_2 washout curves can detect minor degrees of small airway obstruction,[21] but this is a time-consuming and demanding test. The recording of MEFV curves is simple and has a high level of patient acceptance. Its evaluation can now be performed by digital computer.[22] This may yield a suitable quality-controlled routine method for the clinical evaluation of children with chronic respiratory disease such as asthma and cystic fibrosis.

REFERENCES

1. Zapletal, A., Motoyama, E. K., van de Woestijne, K. P., Hunt, V. R., and Bouhuys, A.: Maximum expiratory flow-volume curves and airway conductance in children and adolescents. J. Appl. Physiol., 26:308, 1969.

2. Shwachman, H., and Kulczychi, L. L.: Long-term study of one-hundred-five patients with cystic fibrosis: Studies made over a five to fourteen year period. Amer. J. Dis. Child., 96:6, 1958.

3. Bouhuys, A.: Recent applications of volume displacement body plethysmographs. Progr. Resp. Res., 4:24, 1969.

4. DuBois, A. B., Botelho, S. Y., and Comroe, J. H., Jr.: A new method for measuring airway resistance in man using a body plethysmograph: Values in normal subjects and in patients with respiratory disease. J. Clin. Invest., 35:326, 1956.

5. Bedell, G. N., Marshall, R., DuBois, A. B., and Comroe, J. H., Jr.: Plethysmographic determination of the volume of gas trapped in the lungs. J. Clin. Invest., 35:664, 1956.

6. Milic-Emili, J., Mead, J., Turner, J. M., and Glauser, E. M.: Improved technique for estimat-

ing pleural pressure from esophageal balloons. J. Appl. Physiol., 19:207, 1964.

7. DeMuth, G. R., Howatt, W. F., and Talner, N. S.: Intrapulmonary gas distribution in cystic fibrosis. Amer. J. Dis. Child., 103:129, 1962.

8. Bouhuys, A., Hunt, V. R., Kim, B. M., and Zapletal, A.: Maximum expiratory flow rates in induced bronchoconstriction in man. J. Clin. Invest., 48:1159, 1969.

9. Bouhuys, A.: Airway dynamics and bronchoactive agents in man. In Bouhuys, A., ed.: Airway Dynamics—Physiology and Pharmacology. Springfield, Illinois: Charles C Thomas, p. 263, 1970.

10. Butler, J., Caro, C. G., Alcala, R., and DuBois, A. B.: Physiological factors affecting airway resistance in normal subjects and in patients with obstructive respiratory disease. J. Clin. Invest., 39:584, 1960.

11. Bouhuys, A., and Jonson, B.: Alveolar pressure, airflow rate, and lung inflation in man. J. Appl. Physiol., 22:1086, 1967.

12. Wentworth, P., Gough, J., and Wentworth, J. E.: Pulmonary changes and cor pulmonale in mucoviscidosis. Thorax, 23:582, 1968.

13. Mellins, R. B., Levine, O. R., Ingram, R. H., Jr., and Fishman, A. P.: Obstructive disease of the airways in cystic fibrosis. PEDIATRICS, 141:560, 1968.

14. Bouhuys, A., and van de Woestijne, K. P.: Mechanical consequences of airway smooth muscle relaxation. J. Appl. Physiol., 30:670, 1971.

15. Lifschitz, M. I., and Denning, C. R.: Assessment of bronchospasm in patients with cystic fibrosis. Amer. Rev. Resp. Dis., 99:399, 1969.

16. Motoyama, E. K., Gibson, L. E., Zigas, C. J., and Cook, C. D.: Reevaluation of mist therapy in children with cystic fibrosis using maximum expiratory flow-volume curves. Amer. Ped. Soc./ Soc. Pediat. Res., (Abst.) 101, 1970.

17. Matthews, L. W., Doershuk, C. F., and Spector, S.: Mist tent therapy of the obstructive pulmonary lesion of cystic fibrosis. PEDIATRICS, 39:176, 1967.

18. Emery, J., ed.: The Anatomy of the Developing Lung. Suffolk, England: Lavenham Press Ltd., pp. 15–16, 1969.

19. Bouhuys, A., and van de Woestijne, K. P.: Respiratory mechanics and dust exposure in byssinosis. J. Clin. Invest., 49:106, 1970.

20. Woolcock, A. J., Vincent, N. J., and Macklem, P. T.: Frequency dependence of compliance as a test for obstruction in the small airways. J. Clin. Invest., 48:1097, 1969.

21. Bouhuys, A., Jönsson, R., Lichtneckert, S., Lindell, S.-E., Lundgren, C., Lundin, G., and Ringquist, T. R.: Effects of histamine on pulmonary ventilation in man. Clin. Sci, 19:79, 1960.

22. Bouhuys, A., and Gulesian, P. J.: Electronic data processing of flow and volume data from forced expiratory maneuvers. Amer. Rev. Resp. Dis., 101:1000, 1970.

NEUTRON ACTIVATION ANALYSIS TECHNIQUE FOR NAIL SODIUM CONCENTRATION IN CYSTIC FIBROSIS PATIENTS

G. Frank Johnson, M.D., Max F. Thompson, M.N.E., S. Fetteroff, M.S., and A. N. Fasano, M.C.E

A STUDY has been carried out on the use of neutron activation analysis in the determination of sodium concentration in human nails. The nail samples were obtained from children's hospital patients, cystic fibrosis patients, newborn infants, normal children, normal adults, and from a family with cystic fibrosis in a grandchild. Activation analysis on 111 samples of human nails constitutes the bases of this report.

PURPOSE

The purposes were: (1) to evaluate factors influencing results arising from the use of nails for test objects; (2), to obtain sufficient sampling of normal patients, abnormal patients, and patients with cystic fibrosis to evaluate expected ranges of nail sodium level in health and disease; (3) to establish nail sodium values by neutron activation analysis for future comparisons with an atomic absorption method. The ultimate goal is an accurate method for the neonatal diagnosis of cystic fibrosis using readily available samples suitable for mass screening.

MATERIALS AND METHODS

The majority of the data were obtained from samples not washed or changed in any way before irradiation for 1 hour in a neutron flux of 5×10^{12} n/cm^2-sec, in a nuclear reactor facility. The predominant reaction was the n,γ in that the flux was predominately thermal neutrons. The flux field has been monitored for a period of 4 years and the relative thermal to fast neutron energies in the facility environment have remained constant. The intercomparison of comparator from run to run and the cross correlating with co-foils° were better than a $+1\%$ internal precision. Single nail samples analyzed from four separately generated photopeaks showed similar precision.

The irradiated samples were counted with a 3×3 in. sodium iodide (T^I) detector. A 400 channel analyzer was employed in obtaining the total spectrum of gamma emission from the nail samples. The channel calibration was set at 10 Kev. per channel.

° A co-foil is another metal or compound sample exposed to comparable flux for cross check purposes.

The total spectrum was analyzed for possible interference to the 2.75 Mev. gamma emitted by Na²⁴. It was found that this photopeak was free of interference from chlorine and potassium. The 2.75 Mev. photopeak count is the only part of the spectrum used for the analysis.

These samples were compared to measured quantities of Na₂ Co₃ exposed to the same neutron flux environment along with cobalt wires for interexposure correlation. The sodium carbonate standard was used as a comparator to minimize radioactivity of the standard. This was justified in that the 2.75 Mev. peak area was being used for comparison and analysis of the sodium concentration. The lack of other constituents such as potassium and chlorine did not alter the reliability of the comparator technique. The net results of adding these constituents would raise the total count level and affect the dead time of the counter. Tests showed that 40% dead times could be handled with no error to the 2.75 Mev. photopeak counts.

TABLE I

SODIUM CONCENTRATION IN 111 NAIL SAMPLES

Data	Fingernails	Toenails
	(Mean Na mEq/kg)	
Normal		
29 newborn infants	101.76±21.6	
35 children		
male	58±12.8	73±15.5
female	58± 8.2	72±10
23 adults		
male	32± 4.3	40± 5.9
female	20± 4.9	38± 9.3
cystic fibrosis children		
male		267±24.3
female		261±42.5

A geometrical correction factor was determined to allow comparison between the Na₂ Co₃ samples and the nail samples. This correction was 0.970 when a 1 ml of Na₂ Co₃ water solution was compared to a Na₂ Co₃ precipitate deposited onto an aluminum foil simulating a nail sample. This allowed

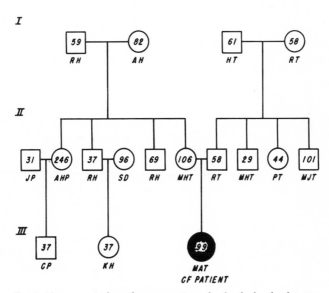

FIG. 1. Measurements from three generations of a family for the detection of heterozygotes in cystic fibrosis.

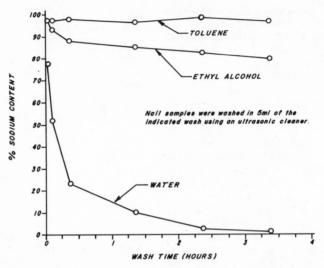

Fig. 2. Washing experiment on nails using organic and inorganic solvents.

for the absolute determination of sodium in the nail sample.

The $Na_2 Co_3$ samples ranged from 0.516 to 51.62 μg of sodium per milliliter of water. Comparator samples weights were chosen according to the report of Gareis and Anderson,[1] whose results showed a range of sodium from 1.8 ± 0.13 to 70.4 ± 1.7 mEq/ kg of fingernail.

RESULTS

Four separate series of experimental determinations were performed. The summary values are presented in Table I.

A separate study of 17 nail sodium determination on three generations of a family in whom a cystic fibrosis patient was present is shown in Figure 1.

DISCUSSION

Age of the patient is clearly an important factor in the level of nail sodium. Normal infants have a high average sodium nail content. Normal newborn infants in this series had nail sodium levels of 101.76 mEq/

kg $\pm$ 21.6. This indicates a need for a separate newborn diagnostic index from the 110 mEq/kg in toenails recommended by Stamm, Woodruff, and Babb[2]† as an index level for separating C. F. patients from normals. The relationship of sodium content of newborns' nails to their fluid environment and the rate of change of sodium nail levels in the neonatal period are now being studied.

A second important factor in evaluation of the results is the site from which the nail sample is obtained. Inorganic sodium salts, not removed by organic solvents (Fig. 2), are absorbed into the nails, and the concentration of sweat around the nail will affect its sodium level, as will its thickness. Data in Table I indicates that the toenail sodium concentration is consistently higher than that found in fingernails in contrast to the results of two other studies.[3,4]

Figure 3 indicates that sodium absorption in nail samples *in vitro* is a function of time

---

† Newborn standard indicated.

122

and sodium concentration, with more rapid absorption by toenails than fingernails, and partial equilibrium after 4 hours of exposure to 7.2 mEq/liter. When nail samples were washed, a state of equilibrium was approached in 3 hours. This would imply extraction of over 95% of the sodium (Fig. 2). The practical significance of this in relation to the effects of swimming has been previously pointed out by others.[5]

An additional factor influencing nail sodium is the state of emotion or health of the patient. Figure 4 indicates the higher concentration of nail sodium in sick than in well people, with a considerable overlap of values from cystic fibrosis and non cystic fibrosis patients. The overlap values be-

tween the latter group might be expected from studies of Landing and Wells[6] on the basic anatomy of eccrine sweat glands in which normal eccrine glands occurred in only 7 of 39 genetic and other diseases classified by proportions of secretory coils and excretory ducts. The known influences of thermal, emotional, and medication factors on sweat physiology are beyond the scope of these comments, but they are believed to explain the distribution patterns in the hospitalized population.

The data of Figure 1 indicate the asymptomatic and presumably heterozygote parent may have nail sodium levels as high as the symptomatic homozygote patient. Schwachman and Kopito[7] had previ-

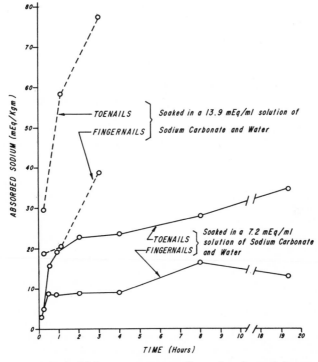

Fig. 3. Sodium solubility curves comparing fingernails and toenails by concentrations.

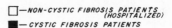

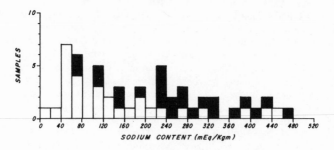

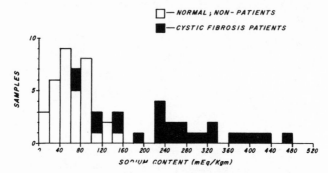

FIG. 4. Summary graph comparing sodium values in hospitalized patients versus cystic fibrosis; and normal versus cystic fibrosis patients.

ously concluded the parents of cystic fibrosis patients could not be distinguished by nail sodium analysis.

amniotic fluid obtained by amniocentesis, may provide valuable earlier measurements of neonatal sodium levels.

SPECULATION AND RELEVANCE

This study provides supportive data for other reports on the practical use of neutron activation techniques in nail sodium determinations. For large sample surveys, to detect cystic fibrosis in newborn infants more practical methods of analysis such as atomic absorption are suggested. The data of this report should be useful in evaluating even more simple analysis techniques. Nail sodium offers an indirect measurement influenced by extrinsic values. Continued research on other test materials, including

SUMMARY

This report describes determination of nail sodium concentration by neutron activation analysis. Results of 111 analyses are summarized by age, sex, normal patients, and abnormal patients. The elevated level of sodium in cystic fibrosis is clearly indicated by this method. Although discussion of results indicates variations associated with age, other illnesses, and factors influencing nail environment, the method may be useful in screening infants for cystic fibrosis.

Less expensive and demanding techniques are being studied.

REFERENCES

1. Gareis, F. J., and Anderson, G. H.: The possible detection of cystic fibrosis by means of the neutron-activation analysis of fingernails. Trans. Amer. Nucl. Soc., 10:57, 1967.
2. Stamm, S. J., Woodruff, G. L., and Babb, A. L.: Cystic fibrosis screening by neutron activation analysis. Cystic Fibrosis Club Abstracts, April 29, 1969, p. 22.
3. Antonelli, M., Ballati, G., and Annibaldi, L.: Simplified nail clipping test for diagnosis of cystic fibrosis. Arch. Dis. Child., 44:218, 1969.
4. Kopito, L., Mahmoodian, A., Townley, R. R. W., Khaw, K. T., and Shwachman, H.: Studies in cystic fibrosis: Analysis of nail clippings for sodium and potassium. New Eng. J. Med., 272:504, 1965.
5. Woodruff, G. L. Wilson, W. E., Jr., Yamamoto, Y., Babb, A. L. and Stamm, S. J.: Clinical experience with the use of neutron activation analysis in the diagnosis of cystic fibrosis. Third International Conference on Modern Trends in Activation Analysis. Gaithersburg, Maryland, October 7–11, 1968, p. 156.
6. Landing, B. H., and Wells, T. R.: Sweat gland anatomy in genetic diseases. J. Chron. Dis., 21:703, 1969.
7. Shwachman, H. and Kopito, L.: Some genetic considerations in cystic fibrosis. A study of nail and sweat sodium in two sibships. Acta Paediat. Scand. (Suppl.), 172:192, 1967.

Diagnosis of Cystic Fibrosis

SIR,—Your leading article (28 August, p. 489) regarding the diagnosis of cystic fibrosis mentions that a simple test of the albumin content of meconium may prove useful in screening for cystic fibrosis at birth.

If such a test is used it must be clearly understood that a proportion of patients with cystic fibrosis have no clinical evidence of malabsorption (approximately 10-15%) and that such cases may not show a positive meconium test.

We have recently seen one such false negative case. Meconium from the day old sister of a child with cystic fibrosis was tested according to the Green and Schwachman technique[1] and gave a normal result. Later sweat tests, however, showed elevated sodium and chloride and the infant was proved to have cystic fibrosis, but without significant malabsorption. She responded well to antibiotic and physiotherapy for any pulmonary problems but did not require pancreatic enzyme replacement.—We are, etc.,

A. G. F. DAVIDSON
CHARLOTTE M. ANDERSON

[1] Green, M. N., and Schwachman, H., *Pediatrics*, 1968, **41**, 989.

Therapy

EVALUATION OF MIST TENT THERAPY IN CYSTIC FIBROSIS USING MAXIMUM EXPIRATORY FLOW VOLUME CURVE

E. K. Motoyama, M.D., L. E. Gibson, M.D., and C. J. Zigas

M IST therapy has been used empirically for many years and has enjoyed wide acceptance in the United States. Currently the use of a mist tent is recommended as an integral part in the treatment of cystic fibrosis both during hospitalization and at home.[1] The rationale for such mist tent therapy in cystic fibrosis is based on the assumption that it provides deposition of small water particles in the lower respiratory tract which in turn liquify tenacious mucus and facilitate its removal.[2] Thus, home mist tent therapy is thought both to prevent and treat obstructive lung disease in cystic fibrosis patients.[2,3]

The wide-spread acceptance of mist tent therapy occurred despite the fact that only one group has presented evidence of its beneficial effects on ventilatory function;[2,3] more recent studies by others have failed to produce similar results.[4,5] Since mist tent therapy is not innocuous,[6,7] the present investigation was undertaken to reexamine its effect on lower airway obstruction in cystic fibrosis.

MATERIAL AND METHODS

The patients with cystic fibrosis (10 boys, six girls; 8 to 15 years of age) included in this study were under the care of the Cystic Fibrosis Clinic at Yale-New Haven Medical Center. The diagnosis was established by

---

Abbreviations

FEV_1: Forced expiratory volume at one second

FRC: Functional residual capacity

Gaw: Airway conductance

MBC: Maximum breathing capacity

MEFV: Maximum expiratory flow volume

PEFR: Peak expiration flow rate

RV: Residual volume

TLC: Total lung capacity

VC: Vital capacity

$\dot{V}max$: Maximum expiratory flow rates measured on MEFV curves

---

This work was supported in part by U. S. Public Health Service Grants HE-14179, HD-03119, by the National Cystic Fibrosis Research Foundation, and by the Health Department of the State of Connecticut.

TABLE I

Comparison of the Mean Ventilatory Function Values During the
Period on versus the Period Off Mist Tent Therapy

	VC	FEV_1	$\dot{V}$ max $(50\% \, VC)$	$\dot{V}$ max $(25\% \, VC)$
Number of patients	16	16	16	16
Off mist tent (% predicted ± S.E.)	89.9±5.3	74.5±4.7	58.7±6.9	46.1±7.7
On mist tent (% predicted ± S.E.)	86.6±4.5	70.9±4.5	52.4±7.4	33.1±7.2
Off mist/on mist (% ± S.E.)	101.8±5.3	105.3±2.1	113.3±6.1	128.0±8.9
Significance	p>0.5	p<0.025	p<0.1	p<0.05

clinical criteria, sweat tests, and radiological findings. The clinical condition of the patient was scored according to the criteria of Shwachman and Kulczycki.[8] The average score of the group was 74 (range, 50 to 90). All of the patients had slept in a mist tent for 6 months or more prior to the study. Fourteen patients used a jet type nebulizer* while two used an ultrasonic nebulizer.† Either tap water or distilled water was used in the nebulizer. Propylene glycol was not added.

In these children ventilatory function studies were repeated every 2 weeks. The study lasted 4 to 5 months during the summer and fall when the absolute humidity in the atmosphere was relatively high. Ventilatory function studies consisted of the measurement of maximum expiratory flow volume (MEFV) curves, forced expiratory volume at 1 second (FEV_1), and vital capacity (VC). All studies were performed and ventilatory function values recorded by the same person who had no knowledge of the method of treatment.

MEFV curves were obtained with a mechanical flow-volume device similar to the one described by Peters, et al.[9] but modified for use in children. During a forced expiration to residual volume (RV) preceded by a full inspiration to total lung capacity (TLC), flow and volume signals were fed into the X and Y axis of the device and the flow-volume curve was mechanically drawn on a 3×5 in. index card. At least three satisfactory MEFV curves were obtained and the curve which had the largest VC was used for analysis. Maximum expiratory flow rates ($\dot{V}$max) at 50% and 25% of VC were measured from

MEFV curves as described elsewhere.[10] FEV_1 was measured at least 3 times using a Collins 6 liter Vitalometer‡ and was expressed in absolute volume as well as percent of VC. VC was measured both from MEFV curves and from Vitalometer readings and the larger volume was recorded when there were discrepancies between the two. Volumes measured were corrected to body temperature (BTPS).

The patients were divided into two groups of eight each. In the first group, studies were made during the initial period of 8 to 10 weeks when they were *off* mist tent therapy. Studies were continued for a similar period after the children were back *on* mist every night. In the second group of eight children the test conditions were reversed. An average of eight studies were performed in each patient. Except for occasional upper respiratory infections, the patient's condition was stable during the study periods. Those who failed to sleep in the mist tent consistently during the study period have been excluded from the present investigation.

In conjunction with the present study, home visits were made to ascertain the amount of contamination of the mist equipment. Prior to the visit the families were asked to leave the water from the previous night in the reservoir so that the operation of the equipment could be observed. Samples

---

* Winliz Floating Island Nebulizer; Winliz Instrumentation, Ltd., Scarborough, Ontario. Canada.

† Mistogen Ultrasonic Nebulizer, Model: EN-140; Mistogen Co., Oakland, California.

‡ W. E. Colleirs, Inc., Braentree Massachusetts.

of water in the nebulizer reservoir, swabbings of the tent wall, and 10-minute fallout in the tent were cultured in order to detect bacterial contamination. Information on frequency of cleaning the equipment was obtained from the parents.

RESULTS

During the entire period of the study the clinical score (8) of 16 patients involved in this study did not change significantly.

The ventilatory function study involving MEFV curves and FEV_1 usually took less than 10 minutes during an outpatient visit. Ventilatory function values obtained from individuals often exhibited variations from one visit to the next; therefore, all values for each test were averaged for each patient for the period on mist and compared with the average values during the period off mist. The data obtained from the two groups (i.e., those on then off mist, and those off then on) were pooled for statistical analysis since no significant difference was found between the two. The results were expressed as percent of the values predicted on the basis of height as previously obtained in our laboratory.[10] Table I. shows the mean values ($\pm SE$) of VC, FEV_1, $\dot{V}max$ (50% VC), and $\dot{V}max$ (25% VC) on versus off mist tent expressed as percent of values predicted on the basis of height. Figures 1, 2, 3, and 4 compare the mean values of VC, FEV_1, $\dot{V}max$ (50% VC), and $\dot{V}max$ (25% VC) respectively on versus off mist tent in each individual. These data show no evidence of improvement but a trend of slight deterioration associated with the use of home mist tent. In particular, the mean values of FEV_1, and $\dot{V}max$ at 25% VC were significantly lower when the patients were on than when they were off mist tent.

Cultures obtained from home mist tent equipment showed that 47% of the tent walls, 80% of water in the nebulizer reservoirs, and 67% of 10 minute fallout in the tent were contaminated with various organisms including *Pseudomonas aeruginosa* and *Escherichia coli*. The parents of these patients had all been given written instructions to clean the tents and nebulizers at least weekly

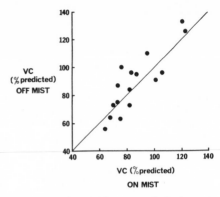

FIG. 1. Comparison of VC on versus off mist therapy in each patient with cystic fibrosis. Each filled circle compares the two mean VC values expressed as percent of predicted values in each patient. A 45° line is the line of identity (i.e., values fall on this line if the mean values on and off mist tent therapy are identical). Those above the line indicate that the mean VC is higher while the patients were off than on mist. There is no difference between the two means. See text.

with a 5% solution of vinegar in water (approximately 0.25% acetic acid solution).[11] In addition, the importance of such cleaning had repeatedly been emphasized during clinic visits. The survey revealed a variation in the

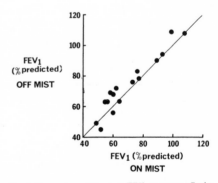

FIG. 2. Comparison of the mean FEV_1 on versus off mist therapy in each patient with cystic fibrosis. A 45° line is the line of identity. The filled circles above the line indicate that the mean FEV_1 is higher while the patients were off than on mist. On paired t-test the mean FEV_1 off mist is significantly ($p < 0.025$) higher than that on mist. See text.

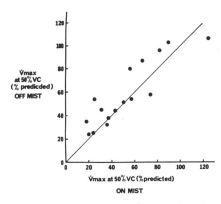

Vmax
at 50% VC
(% predicded)
OFF MIST

Vmax at 50% VC (% predicted)

ON MIST

FIG. 3. Comparison of the mean V̇max at 50% VC on versus off mist therapy in each patient with cystic fibrosis. A 45° line is the line of identity. The filled circles above the line indicate that the mean V̇max is higher while the patients were off than on mist. There is a tendency for the mean V̇max *off* mist to be higher than V̇max on mist (p < 0.1). See text.

frequency of cleaning from daily to never. There was, however, no apparent correlation between the frequency of cleaning and contamination.

DISCUSSION

Present studies of serial ventilatory function tests in patients with mild to moderate cystic fibrosis failed to demonstrate any beneficial effects of mist tent therapy. Moreover, during the period when these patients were off mist therapy at night, their ventilatory function tended to improve slightly while the clinical scores did not alter significantly. These results disagree with the reports of Matthews, Doershuk, and their associates[2,3] in which mist tent therapy was found to be beneficial. The discrepancy between the two groups of studies may in part be due to the selection of ventilatory function tests since the efficacy of mist tent therapy in children with cystic fibrosis can only be evaluated with appropriate tests of ventilatory function. First, such ventilatory function tests should be specifically sensitive for detecting lower airway obstruction as it is one of the main features of the ventilatory

problems in this disease.[12] Second, the test should be reproducible and influenced as little as possible by effort so that the result is not affected by the patient's psychological and emotional state. Finally, such a test should be simple to perform, of short duration and require minimum cooperation, particularly for young children.

In the previous studies[5] in children with mild airway obstruction, we compared the relative sensitivity of various ventilatory function tests including total lung capacity (TLC), vital capacity (VC), functional residual capacity/total lung capacity (FRC/TLC) ratio using both the helium dilution technique and a body plethysmograph, forced expiratory volume at 1 second (FEV$_1$), peak flow rate (PEFR), airway conductance (Gaw), and maximum expiratory flow rates (V̇max) at 50% and 25% of VC on maximum expiratory flow-volume (MEFV) curve. We found that the measurement of V̇max was by far the most sensitive test for lower airway obstruction. In 28 patients with cystic fibrosis about 70% of them showed significantly abnormal values (i.e., more than 2 SD below the predicted values) of V̇max at 25% VC although their VC and TLC were in most cases within normal limits. Among the conventional tests of ventilatory capacity, the measurement of FEV$_1$ was superior to others; about 40% of the same group of patients showed significantly abnormal values. Other tests were less sensitive for the detection of airway obstruction. These data are in agreement with the recent report by Featherby, *et al.*[12]

Unlike conventional tests for ventilatory capacity which measure the relationship between the volume and time, MEFV curve relates maximum expiratory flow-rates (V̇max) to corresponding lung volumes during forced expiration.[14] One of the important features of this measurement is that at lower lung volumes (i.e., less than 60 to 70% of VC) V̇max is, to a considerable extent, independent of the degree of expiratory effort and is readily reproducible. This effort independence of V̇max is the result of the dynamic compression of relatively large intra-

131

thoracic airways. Vmax thus becomes independent of changes in upper airway resistance and is determined by the static recoil pressure of the lung and flow resistance of lower airways upstream from the segment of dynamic compression.[15] Since the static recoil pressure of the lung is within normal limits in children with cystic fibrosis with mild to moderate airway obstruction,[5] Vmax reflects changes in lower airway resistance (or changes proportional to lower airway conductance) where the pathological changes of cystic fibrosis take place.[12] It is preferable to measure MEFV curves with a body plethysmograph so that Vmax can be expressed at certain thoracic gas volumes (i.e., 50% TLC) regardless of changes in VC or RV. However, a simple mechanical flow-volume device was used in the present studies since one purpose of the study was to establish a simple yet sensitive method for assessing lower airway obstruction which can be used in pediatric outpatient clinics or in hospitals without highly specialized pulmonary function laboratories. In addition, it was not practical to study these young patients in a body plethysmograph every two weeks. In order to minimize the artifactual changes in Vmax due to changes in VC, the largest VC for each patient during the course of the study was used to standardize the values of his 50% VC and 25% VC since it was found that the changes in VC in patients with cystic fibrosis were primarily due to changes in RV, rather than changes in TLC.[5]

In their studies of mist tent therapy, Matthews, Doershuk, and their associates[2,3] measured VC, FRC, RV, RV/TLC ratio, and MBC (maximum breathing capacity). Tests such as PEFR, RV, and MBC are heavily dependent on the patient's effort and muscle strength.[16] These effort-dependent tests can therefore be influenced by psychological and emotional states of patients; thus, evaluation of the result is difficult. Measurement of FRC and calculation of the FRC/TLC ratio or RV/TLC ratio are sensitive provided that FRC is obtained with a body plethysmograph (FRC_{box}). In

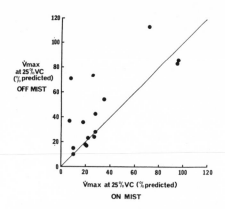

FIG. 4. Comparison of the mean Vmax at 25% VC on versus off mist therapy in each patient with cystic fibrosis. A 45° line is the line of identity. The filled circle above the line indicates that the mean Vmax is higher while the patients were off than on mist. On paired t-test the mean Vmax at 25% VC is significantly (p < <0.05) higher than the mean on mist. See text.

patients with airway obstruction, however, the measurement of FRC with the conventional helium dilution method (FRC_{He}) gives falsely low values and may be misleading.[5,13,17] The difference between FRC_{box} and FRC_{He} is the amount of trapped air in the lungs.[5] Indeed, in the previous studies improvement of airway obstruction in patients evidenced by a decrease in true FRC (FRC_{box}) was often associated with a paradoxical increase in FRC_{He}. The latter increase is apparently the result of the reopening of obstructed airways.

The present studies point out the necessity of serial and specific pulmonary function studies at relatively short intervals in patients with cystic fibrosis in order to evaluate such therapy as mist. Since there are day today or week-to-week fluctuations of ventilatory function in these patients, a comparison of a single determination of pulmonary function with versus without mist may be misleading.

The case for mist tent therapy must be examined carefully since the tratment is not without complications.[6,8] Bacterial contamination, particularly with *Pseudomonas aeruginosa,* is a constant hazard as shown in this study as well as by others[18] even with daily cleaning with 0.25% acetic acid.[11] The lack of correlation between the frequency of cleaning the mist tent apparatus and the incidence of bacterial contamination in the present series merely adds to the already abundant evidence indicating the near impossibility of keeping home mist tents uncontaminated. Indeed, as pointed out by Grieble, *et al.,*[19] nothing short of daily sterilization with ethylene oxide or other means, and the use of sterile water, all of which are impractical with home therapy, is likely to solve this problem. We speculate, although it is impossible to prove, that the small but significant decreases in ventilatory function observed with the use of mist tent in the present study may in part be related to bacterial contamination of equipment and increased pulmonary infection.

The deterioration in pulmonary function noted in this study may also be the result of bronchospasm produced by inhalation of mist.[20-23] In bronchitic patients bronchospasm thus produced was often associated with significant decreases in arterial oxygen tensions.[23] Chronic exposure to ultrasonically produced mist in dogs produced progressive atelectasis, increased intrapulmonary shunt, and the lesions compatible with severe bronchopneumonia.[24] Furthermore, in small infants mist may create additional hazards of over-hydration and disturbances in body temperature regulation by evaporation.[6]

Indirect evidence on the inefficacy of mist tent therapy was presented in the recent studies by Wolfsdorf, Swift and Avery,[25] and by Aspin, *et al.*[26] These authors utilized radioactive technetium-tagged mist and could not demonstrate any significant deposition of water below the larynx during normal nasal or mouth breathing. Neither distilled water or a mixture of 10% propylene glycol in water[2] was deposited in the lower respiratory tracts. These findings, however, do not exclude the possible therapeutic effect of mist therapy for upper airway disease (such as epiglottitis or tracheitis) or of intermittent aerosol therapy via a mouth tube since more water can be deposited beyond the larnyx with tube breathing.[25] The present series did not include patients with severe cases of cystic fibrosis and, therefore, further studies are necessary to rule out the possibility that such patients may benefit from the mist.

Mist tent may be beneficial by preventing evaporation from the upper airways as recently proposed by Matthews.[27] The effect of "hydration of airways" needs to be evaluated carefully.[28] Present studies were performed during the summer and fall, when atmospheric humidity was relatively high, to avoid the possible harmful effect of breathing dry air. If the prevention of upper airway dehydration is the objective, oral hydration of the patient[25] together with the use of a heated humidifier for the entire room may be a safer and easier alternative for mist tent therapy since there is far less danger of bacterial contamination with a humidifier which generates bacteria-free water vapor.

Studies by Dooley[29] on the life span of patients with cystic fibrosis failed to show significant overall prolongation of survival of such pateints after the introduction of home mist tent therapy while other forms of therapy remained unchanged. He attributed the recent improvement in survival of children with cystic fibrosis not to mist but to a number of factors, particularly the development of regional cystic fibrosis centers for continuous care of patients as well as the more liberal use of antibotics. Warwick[30] demonstrated the recent improvement in survival of patients with cystic fibrosis, particularly among the patients of Matthews and his associates.[27] This finding is often cited as evidence for mist tent therapy, but as pointed out by Dooley[29] this improvement in life expectancy may be attributed to excellent overall patient care rather than the effect of mist tent therapy per se.

Proponents of mist tent therapy may object that there were too few patients, a too short study period, and less than optimal mist generations in the present study. It is difficult to refute all of these arguments. The present report, although involving only 16 patients, is based on over 130 separate series of ventilatory function studies. The study period of 4 to 5 months may be short but was used in the previous studies[2,3] to show changes in pulmonary function in cystic fibrosis patients. Both types of nebulizers used in the present study produce relatively high mist output. Although the mass median diameter of water particles and mist density may differ between the two, the result from those who used supposedly more effective ultrasonic nebulizers in the present study did not differ from those who used Winliz (jet type) nebulizers. Certainly, some patients may be improved with some type of mist therapy for some period of time. The authors can only say that, on the basis of their studies and the current literature, they can not identify such patients.

SPECULATION AND RELEVANCE

Mist tent therapy is widely used, especially in the treatment of cystic fibrosis. It is expensive, unpleasant, and possibly hazardous. There is good evidence that little water is delivered to the lungs. The present study shows no benefit of nocturnal mist tent therapy for the cystic fibrosis patients studied. In view of these data the authors recommend that, except for further controlled studies, the use of mist tent for the treatment of lower respiratory tract disease such as cystic fibrosis, bronchiolitis, and pneumonia be discontinued.

SUMMARY

Using primarily maximum expiratory-flow-volume curves, a simple but highly sensitive test for evaluating lower airway obstruction, the efficacy of nocturnal mist tent therapy was evaluated in 16 patients with cystic fibrosis every two weeks for 4 to 5 months when they were on and off mist tent therapy.

No evidence of improvement was found in ventilatory function of these patients with mist tent therapy. On the contrary, there was evidence of small but significant decreases in ventilatory function of these patients during the period when they were on mist tent therapy.

REFERENCES

1. Guide to Diagnosis and Management of Cystic Fibrosis. New York: National Cystic Fibrosis Research Foundation, 1963.
2. Matthews, L. W., Doershuk, C. F., and Spector, S.: Mist tent therapy of the obstructive pulmonary lesion of cystic fibrosis. PEDIATRICS, 39:176, 1967.
3. Doershuk, C. F., Matthews, L. W., Gillespie, C. T., Lough, M. D., and Spector, S.: Evaluation of jet-type and ultrasonic nebulizers in mist tent therapy for cystic fibrosis. PEDIATRICS, 41:723, 1968.
4. Norman, A. P.: In Discussion on Therapeutic and Prophylactic Use of Mist Tents. Fifth International Cystic Fibrosis Conference, Cambridge, September 22–26, 1969, p. 151, Cystic Fibrosis Research Trust.
5. Zapletal, A., Motoyama, E. K., Gibson, L. E., and Bouhuys, A.: Pulmonary mechanics in asthma and cystic fibrosis. PEDIATRICS, 48:64, 1971.
6. Avery, M. E., Galina, M., and Nachman, R.: Mist therapy. PEDIATRICS, 39:160, 1967.
7. Graff, T. D., and Benson, D. W.: Systemic and pulmonary changes with inhaled humid atmospheres: Clinical application. Anesthesiology, 30:199, 1969.
8. Shwachman, H., and Kulczycki, L. L.: Long-term study of one hundred five patients with cystic fibrosis: Studies made over a five to fourteen year period. Amer. J. Dis. Child, 96:6, 1958.
9. Peters, J. M., Mead, J., and VanGanse, W. F.: A simple flow-volume device for measuring ventilatory function in the field. Amer. Rev. Resp. Dis., 99:617, 1969.
10. Zapletal, A., Motoyama, E. K., Van d. Woestijne, K. P., Hunt, V. R., and Bouhuys, A.: Maximum expiratory flow-volume curves and airway conductance in children and adolescents. J. Appl. Physiol., 26:308, 1969.
11. Pierce, A. K., Sanford, J. P., Thomas, G. D., and Leonard, J. S.: Long-term evaluation of decontamination of inhalation-therapy equipment and the occurrence of necrotizing pneumonia. New Eng. J. Med., 282:528, 1970.
12. Mellins, R. B.: The site of airway obstruction in cystic fibrosis. PEDIATRICS, 44:315, 1969.
13. Featherby, E. A., Weng, T. R., Crozier, D. N., Duic, A., Reilly, B. J., and Levison, H.: Dynamic and static lung volumes, blood gas tensions, and diffusing capacity in patients with cystic fibrosis. Amer. Rev. Resp. Dis., 102:737, 1970.
14. Fry, D. L., and Hyatt, R. E.: Pulmonary mechanics: A unified analysis of the relationship between

pressure, volume and gas flow in the lungs of normal and diseased human subjects. Amer. J. Med., 29:672, 1960.

15. Mead, J., Turner, J. M., Macklem, P. T., and Little, J. B.: Significance of the relationship between lung recoil and maximum expiratory flow. J. Appl. Physiol., 22:95, 1967.

16. Hyatt, R. E.: Dynamic lung volumes. *In* Fenn, W. O., and Rahn, H., ed.: Handbook of Physiology, Sect. 3, Respiration Vol. 2. Washington, D. C.: American Physiology Society, chapter 54, 1965.

17. Beier, F. R., Renzetti, A. D., Jr., Mitchell, M., and Watanabe, S.: Pulmonary pathophysiology in cystic fibrosis. Amer. Rev. Resp. Dis., 94:430, 1966.

18. Moffet, H. K., and Allan, D.: Colonization of infants exposed to bacterially contaminated mists. Amer. J. Dis. Child, 114:21, 1967.

19. Grieble, H. G., Colton, F. R., Bird, T. J., Toigo, A., and Griffith, L. G.: Fine-particle humidifiers. Source of Pseudomonas aeruginosa infection in a respiratory-disease unit. New Eng. J. Med., 282:531, 1970.

20. Cheney, F. W., and Butler, J.: The effects of ultrasonically-produced aerosols on airway resistance in man. Anesthesiology, 29:1099, 1968.

21. Cheney, F. W., and Butler, J.: The effect of ultrasonic aerosols on the total respiratory resistance of the intubated patient Anesthesiology, 32:456, 1970.

22. Abernethy, J. D.: Effects of inhalation of an artificial fog. Thorax, 23:421, 1968.

23. Pflug, A. E., Cheney, F. W., Jr., and Butler, J.: The effect of an ultrasonic aerosol on pulmonary mechanics and arterial blood gases in patients with chronic bronchitis. Amer. Rev. Resp. Dis., 101:710, 1970.

24. Modell, J. H.: Experimental studies in chronic exposure to ultrasonic nebulized aerosols. J. Asthma Res., 5:223, 1968.

25. Wolfsdorf, J., Swift, D. L., and Avery, M. E.: Mist therapy reconsidered; an evaluation of the respiratory deposition on labelled water aerosols produced by jet and ultrasonic nebulizers. PEDIATRICS, 43:799, 1969.

26. Aspin, N., Bau, S. K., Levison, H., and Wood, D. E.: The distribution of fluid intake from mist tent therapy. (Abst.) Amer. Ped. Soc./Soc. Ped. Res. p. 105, 1970.

27. Matthews, L. W.: *In* Discussion on Therapeutic and Prophylactic Use of Mist Tents. Fifth International Cystic Fibrosis Conference, Cambridge, September 22–26, 1969, p. 155. Cystic Fibrosis Research Trust.

28. Avery, M. E.: *In* Discussion on Therapeutic and Prophylactic Use of Mist Tents. Fifth International Cystic Fibrosis Conference, Cambridge, September 22–26, 1969, p. 165, Cystic Fibrosis Research Trust.

29. Dooley, R. R.: Effect of survival of cystic fibrosis patients by the introduction of home mist tent therapy as measured by the life table. Cystic Fibrosis Club abstract. 11th Annual Meeting, April 29, 1970, Atlantic City, p. 22.

30. Warwick, W. J.: Cystic fibrosis: nature and prognosis. Minn. Med., 50:1049, 1967.

Acknowledgment

The authors are indebted to Dr. Charles D. Cook for his helpful comments.

Buffered L-Arginine as Treatment for Cystic Fibrosis: State of the Evidence

TO THE EDITOR:

Solomons, *et al.* (PEDIATRICS, **47**:384) describe some provocative results with buffered L-arginine in the treatment of cystic fibrosis. In their first paragraph they ascribe, without reference, some fascinating pharmacologic actions to this amino acid. Perhaps they are the result of the most unusual structure, with a supercharged nitrogen, of the arginine they used, so different from the one to which we are accustomed.

In the pulmonary function studies one is disturbed by the fact that both the patients and the individuals administering the aerosol, and presumably promoting the deep breaths, were well aware of the fact that they were using the agent with expected therapeutic effects. Despite previous failures with isotonic saline and urea it might have been wise to use, for the "control," an isotonic solution, perhaps of some more "inert" amino acid. It would be reassuring to know that the studies of pulmonary function were carried out by someone who was unaware of the treatment status and at a time unrelated to the therapeutic sessions. The authors state that "the sputum appeared to be less viscous:" without actual measurements it is difficult to accept such a claim. The disappearance of *Hemophilus* and *Staph. aureus* from the sputum cultures is of interest. If the specimens were obtained immediately after a therapeutic session, might not the high concentration of arginine have inhibited their growth on the culture media?

In the fat absorption studies there was no control over fat intake: without this it is impossible to interpret the results presented. The difficulty is compounded by the absence of an adequate "control" agent, perhaps again another amino acid. The statement is made that "weight gain was well correlated to the de-crease in fecal fat excretion." I plotted one against the other and no such relation was apparent, even when I made a crude correction for age and size in the rates of weight gain. The authors claim that arginine in their studies decreased fecal fat to a greater extent than bicarbonate in the studies of others. Such a comparison hardly seems justifiable.

It would indeed be gratifying if the results obtained were to be confirmed in a properly controlled situation. Until such time, however, only the most cautious enthusiasm seems to be in order.

GEORGE G. GRAHAM, M.D.

EDITOR'S NOTE: Dr. Solomons comments as follows:

In his letter to the Editor, Dr. Graham has requested information concerning, (i) the properties of arginine, (ii) the adequacy of controls for the inhalation and fat absorbtion studies. In answer to these questions the following can be stated: (i) the properties of arginine discussed in the paper have been documented by Clarke, E. R. and Martell, A. G., J. Inorg. Nucl. Chem., 23:911–926, 1970, and Hardel M., and Hoppe Seyl. Z.: Physiol. Chem., 346:224–228, 1966. The ability of arginine to activate trypsin and lipase is described by Bargoni, N.: Studi Sassaresi Sezione I, 38: 204–212, 1960, and Yamamoto, T., J.: Biochem. Japan, 38:147–155, 1957; (ii) We have done double blind control studies using saline and urea and have found no change as stated on page 385 of our paper. However, we were unable to find any product that had the characteristics of the 5% arginine mixture. If Dr. Graham can suggest an inert amino acid or some solution that has the same physical characteristics as arginine, a double blind study could be carried out. The thoracic gas volume is an objective measurement and is difficult to be measured incorrectly even by a biased observer. The sputum collection was done at the time of the pulmonary functions study. The patient received therapy on arising in the morning which was 1 to 2 hours prior to the sputum collection. From the reported animal studies, arginine does not seem to be retained in the airway for more than 30 minutes. However, we have no explanation for the disappearance of the *Hemophilus* and *Staph. aureus*. The sputum appeared to be less viscid when arginine was given. Since no objective measurements were made, this observation was omitted from the original manuscript: It was inserted on the recommendation of a referee. Dr. Graham makes an unjustified statement when he claims that we found arginine to be superior to bicarbonate "in the studies of others," because, on p. 388, we were careful to insert the phrase "in our experience," when dealing with this topic. With regard to fat absorption, the intake of fat was not quantitatively determined; however, the younger patients (#10–14) had a consistently controlled dietary intake on and off arginine therapy. It is difficult to determine whether there was a primary decrease in steatorrhea in any of the patients since improvement could be secondary to improved pulmonary function. The gain in weight was well correlated with fat absorbtion in nine patients but not in six of the patients; however, no patients in this group lost weight. In 32 patients

presently undergoing study, we have subsequently found that watery diarrhea has been a problem with the majority of patients under 3 months of age and teenagers over 14 years. As a cautionary measure, it should be realized that arginine can cause the ingress of water into gut and lung. However, the presence of diarrhea strengthens the authors' prediction that arginine acts by influencing water, and possibly bile transport. It is significant that patients in this group with diarrhea and abdominal pain and weight loss due to arginine maintained their improved pulmonary function and the diarrhea was diminished by reducing the dosage and then increasing it to the previous level. Dosage is very much dependent on the individual patient's tolerance and response; body mass, although convenient, is probably too crude a basis for calculating dosage.

It must be emphasized that L-arginine is still an experimental drug: It is difficult to obtain large quantities and not all brands are pure. However, the beneficial effects of arginine on some C.F. patients have excited sufficient interest to justify continued study of its mechanism of action in those patients who respond favourably.

This comment gives opportunity to correct the formula for arginine which appeared on page 387 of PEDIATRICS, Volume 47. The formula should be:

$$\text{COOH}-\underset{\underset{\text{NH}_2}{|}}{\overset{\overset{\text{H}}{|}}{\text{C}}}-\text{CH}_2-\text{CH}_2-\text{CH}_2-\underset{}{\overset{\overset{\text{H}}{|}}{\text{N}}}-\underset{\underset{\text{NH}_2}{}}{\overset{\overset{\text{NH}}{||}}{\text{C}}}$$

CLIVE C. SOLOMONS

THE USE OF BUFFERED L-ARGININE IN THE TREATMENT OF CYSTIC FIBROSIS

Clive C. Solomons, Ph.D., Ernest K. Cotton, M.D., Reuben Dubois, M.B., B.S.,
with the assistance of Margo Pinney, R.N., B.S.

THE major symptoms of patients with cystic fibrosis (C.F.) are related to the increased state of aggregation and viscosity of bronchiolar and intestinal secretions.[1] The increased viscosity of mucus in C.F. has been attributed to the secretion of abnormal glycoproteins and a disturbed pattern of ionic constituents.[2] The structure of L-arginine indicated that this molecule possesses the advantage of having a variety of physicochemical properties which could work together to reduce the viscosity of biological secretions. Thus the guanidine group (Fig. 1) of arginine would act to disperse and solubilize macromolecules which are stabilized by hydrogen bonding. The carboxylate group of arginine binds metal ions and could aid in the reduction of viscosity due to divalent ion cross-links. The presence of a neutral trimethylene bridge situated between the polar charged groups enables the molecule to act as a mild detergent, which may aid both in decreasing viscosity and in increasing the emulsification of dietary fat in the intestine.

The purpose of this investigation was twofold: (1) to evaluate the effects of argi-nine administered by ultrasonic nebulization in vital capacity, thoracic gas volume, and arterial Po_2 of C.F. patients with chronic obstructive pulmonary disease; (2) to observe the effects of buffered oral arginine on steatorrhea, abdominal pain, and weight gain in C.F. patients who have minimal or no detectable pulmonary disease.

PATIENTS AND METHODS

Part 1: Pulmonary Function Studies

In the first part of the study, eight patients, age 9 to 12 years, were diagnosed by repeated sweat chloride determinations and exhibited the clinical signs of moderate to severe chronic lung disease (Table I).[13] Repeated evaluations of pulmonary functions had been made on these individuals over the past 2 years. Thoracic gas volume (TGV), vital capacity (VC), and specific conductance (G/FRC) were obtained by using a total body volume plethysmograph[3,4] and were stable in these patients for at least 6 months before this study. Chest x-ray films showed that all the patients were hyperaerated and had extensive infiltrates. Two patients (T.G. and A.S.) had general-

Supported by U.S. Public Health Service grant AM08757-06 from the Division of Arthritis and Metabolic Diseases; FR-69; and the National Cystic Fibrosis Foundation 67869.

138

ized interstitial involvement. Sputum cultures grew Hemophilus, Pseudomonas and Staph. aureus. The partial pressure of oxygen was measured in duplicate in 0.6 cc of heparinized arterial blood using oxygen electrode (type E5046 Radiometer).* Care was taken to treat the patients uniformly during control and test periods with regard to antibiotic therapy and physiotherapy. The arginine solution was made up by adding 0.9 gm of L-arginine free base, to 15 gm L-arginine hydrochloride.† The mixture was dissolved in 300 ml of tap water (final pH 7.4-7.6, 290 milliosmol.) and administered for 3 weeks at a time by ultrasonic nebulizer‡ for 30 minutes, 4 times per day. During this 30-minute period, the patient was encouraged to take as many deep breaths as possible. Since no significant change in lung volumes were previously observed using isotonic saline or isotonic urea, water was used for comparison in this study.

Arginine was administered by inhalation for a period of 3 weeks, followed by 3 weeks of water and another 3 weeks of arginine. The patients were then given arginine continuously. Pulmonary functions were measured weekly and the values for the thoracic gas volume and vital capacity at the end of each period are reported. Representative values for specific conductance and Po_2 during water and arginine treatment are also presented.

As arginine imparts as taste to the aerosol which is not easily duplicated, a double blind study was not undertaken.

Part 2: Fat Absorption Studies

In the second part of this study, 14 patients with proven C.F. whose ages ranged from 1 to 19 years were selected (Table II). All except two (2 and 8) had predominantly gastrointestinal symptoms, were free of cough, had clear chest x-rays, and normal pulmonary function tests. One patient (10) with meconium ileus during the neo-

natal period had undergone partial ileal resection. Seven patients were not on pancreatic enzyme supplementation during the period of study. One patient (14a, 14b) was studied both with and without pancrelipase (Cotazym) administration. Nine individuals had recurrent crampy abdominal pain of varying degrees of severity accom-

* Radiometer, Copenhagen, Denmark.
† Sigma Chemical Co., St. Louis, Missouri.
‡ The Monaghan Co., Denver, Colorado.

TABLE I

PATIENTS SELECTED FOR INHALATION STUDIES WHO WERE INTERMITTENTLY GIVEN a BUFFERED MIXTURE OF L-ARGININE AND L-ARGININE HYDROCHLORIDE BY ULTRASONIC NEBULIZER

Name	Age (Yr)	Weight (kg)	Height (cm)	Shwachman Kulczycki Score[13]
D.S.	10	16.5	120	50
P.L.	10	18.8	122	25
J.C.	12	28	141	25
S.C.	9	19.6	123	25
J.L.	9	19.5	116	40
T.B.	6	16.7	107	65
T.G.	8	20	117	50
A.S.	12	26.4	137	30

TABLE II

PATIENTS SELECTED FOR FAT ABSORPTION STUDIES WHO WERE GIVEN BUFFERED L-ARGININE 1 GM/KG/DAY BY MOUTH FOR 10 DAYS

	Patient	Age (yr)	Pulmonary Disease	Cotazym*	Abdominal Pain
1	J.Ro.	19	±	+	+
2	J.L.	11	+	+	+
3	N.M.	11	−	−	−
4	R.S.	7	−	+	+
5	R.M.	6	−	+	+
6	B.K.	6	−	−	+
7	J.Rh.	6	−	+	−
8	J.deL.	5	+	+	+
9	D.E.	4	−	−	+
10	R.T.	2	−	−	−
11	J.C.	2	−	−	+
12	M.T.	1½	−	+	−
13	S.Mc.	1½	−	−	+
14a	K.H.	1	−	+	−
14b	K.H.	1	−	−	−

* 16 to 20, 300 mg capsules per day.

139

TABLE III

EFFECT OF INHALATION OF ULTRASONICALLY NEBULIZED TAP WATER AND BUFFERED 5% L-ARGININE SOLUTION ON THORACIC GAS VOLUME AND VITAL CAPACITY IN PATIENTS WITH CYSTIC FIBROSIS

| Patient | Thoracic Gas Volume (ml) | | | | | Vital Capacity (ml) | | | | |
	Control	3 wk Arginine	3 wk H₂O	3 wk Arginine	2 mo Arginine	Control	3 wk Arginine	3 wk H₂O	3 wk Arginine	2 mo Arginine
T.B.	2,780	1,465	2,300	1,815	1,265	330	750	440	500	600
J.C.	3,000	1,470	2,890	1,950	2,090	1,150	1,890	1,260	1,560	1,650
S.C.	2,400	2,090	2,490	2,400	2,240	800	945	800	830	720
J.L.	2,320	1,575	2,090	1,470	1,310	830	1,575	830	1,000	1,000
P.L.	3,515	1,880	2,065	2,160	1,900	500	630	635	910	800
D.S.	2,015	1,215	2,090	1,690	1,780	525	895	545	800	860
T.G.	3,375	1,520	3,240	1,950	1,950	870	1,330	700	910	970
A.S.	3,660	2,490	3,000	2,890	2,680	1,180	1,450	1,250	1,375	1,410
Mean	2,883	1,713	2,520	2,040	1,902	773	1,183	808	986	1,001
	±606	±414	±465	±444	±465	±305	±444	±304	±335	±356
p treated VS control		<0.005	<0.10	<0.005	<0.005		<0.025	<0.50	<0.10	<0.10
Normal range	1,000–2,000					880–1,700				

P values were derived from the student-t distribution.

panied by palpable masses of intestinal contents and had "meconium ileus equivalent."[5] One patient (4) had surgical reduction of an intussusception 1 month before the study. All patients were weighed before and after the period of investigation. A 72-hour stool fat excretion was determined[6] prior to the oral administration of buffered L-arginine. L-arginine free base and L-arginine hydrochloride were mixed in the ratio of 0.9 gm free base to 15 gm of arginine hydrochloride and the powder was given orally in divided doses of 1 gm/kilogram/24 hours with a maximum of 25 gm for 10 days.

The taste of the buffered arginine mixture was unpalatable to normal volunteers but was well tolerated by the patients when taken in chocolate milk or apple sauce. Capsules were used for one patient who found the taste intolerable. All patients consumed a normal diet and were instructed to adhere closely to the same diet during both test and control periods, but no quantitative determinations of fat intake were made. The 72-hour fecal fat excretion was remea-sured starting 7 days after arginine administration was begun.

RESULTS

Part 1: Measurements of Pulmonary Function

Tables III and IV show the changes in pulmonary functions in the treated patients. All of the patients improved during inhalation of buffered arginine and relapsed to their former state during the control periods. Significant improvements were observed in TGV, arterial Po_2, and specific conductance during periods of treatment with arginine. Vital capacity increased and forced expiratory volume/second improved by 10%. Postural drainage was more productive and the sputum appeared to be less viscous. Hemophilus and Staph. aureus disappeared from the sputum cultures, but pseudomonas remained. Blood leukocyte counts remained in the pretreatment range of 8,800 to 21,400/cmm. Clinical improvement in appearance and exercise tolerance was also seen. If arginine was absorbed by inhalation, the amounts were too small to

140

be detected by partition chromatography done on serum and urine.

Part 2: Fat Absorption Studies

Table V shows the changes in 72-hour fecal fat excretion and the weight gain during 10 days of arginine administration. The mean percentage decrease in steatorrhea was 18.3. All patients gained weight with a mean increase of 0.6 ± 0.5 kg. Nine patients had complained of varying degrees of abdominal pain before therapy: all experienced dramatic relief within 24 to 48 hours of ingesting arginine with recurrence of pain following the cessation of therapy. Using paper chromatography, appreciable quantities of arginine were detected in the urine of treated patients but blood levels were not elevated as judged by this technique.

DISCUSSION

It must be emphasized that arginine free base is a caustic substance and should never be administered to a patient without neutralization with arginine hydrochloride as described in the text. Similarly, arginine hydrochloride is acidic and should be neutralized with free base before use. Since arginine is metabolized to urea and ornithine, it should not be given in large doses to patients whose renal function is compromised in any way.

Part 1: Pulmonary Function Studies

The observed increase in arterial P_{O_2} and the decrease in thoracic gas volume could be due to a combination of the mucolytic, calcium binding, and detergent properties ascribed to arginine.

Vital capacity and forced expiratory volume/second increased but this was significant only in the first period of treatment. However, the vital capacity measurements are not as objective as those of thoracic gas volume. The striking initial improvement in vital capacity is thought to be due to the mobilization of obstructive material in the airway. Since the patients already had long standing, irreversible lung damage, the con-

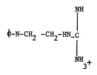

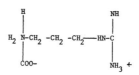

Fig. 1. Formula of arginine and related compounds discussed in the text.

tinued use of arginine did not show further significant improvement. Studies are now in progress on patients with mild to moderate pulmonary involvement in order to evaluate the prophylactic potential of arginine therapy. A pharmocological effect to decrease water reabsorption may have also occurred and this possibility is currently being investigated.

It has been shown *in vitro* that 0.1 gm/ 100 ml arginine will reduce the macromolecular aggregation of tropocollagen molecules, presumably by interfering with hydrogen bonding and charged group interactions. Lysine, in contrast to arginine, greatly enhanced fibril aggregation under these conditions.[7] Arginine has many structural features in common with guanethidine (Fig. 1), a substance which reduced the

TABLE IV

EFFECT OF INHALATION OF BUFFERED 5% ARGININE ON PO2 AND SPECIFIC CONDUCTANCE IN PATIENTS WITH CYSTIC FIBROSIS

Patient	Arterial PO_2 mm Hg Control	Treated	Specific Conductance Control	Treated
T.B.	45	60	0.07	0.33
J.C.	38	50	0.06	0.12
S.C.	28	51	0.09	0.18
J.L.	62	68	0.09	0.17
P.L.	75	85	0.12	0.24
D.S.	45	52	0.10	0.19
T.G.	47	65	0.19	0.29
A.S.	67	76	0.23	0.36
Mean	49 ± 16	63 ± 11	0.13 ± 0.06	0.24 ± 0.08
P	< 0.025		< 0.005	
Normal range	67–76		> 0.2	

P values were derived from the student-t distribution.

turbidy of saliva when given intravenously to C.F. patients.[8] Arginine however, does not have the undesirable side effects on the autonomic sympathetic nervous system

TABLE V

CHANGES IN FECAL FAT AND BODY WEIGHT WHICH ACCOMPANIED THE ORAL ADMINISTRATION OF BUFFERED L-ARGININE 1 gm/KG/DAY FOR 10 DAYS

Patient	Weight Gain (kg)	Fecal Fat Control	gm per 72 hours Treated	% Decrease Steatorrhea
1 J.Ro.	2.2	117	87	26
2 J.L.	0.8	116	107	8
3 N.M.	0.5	184	131	29
4 R.S.	0.6	92	54	41
5 R.M.	0.3	39	39	0
6 B.K.	0.9	41	31	25
7 J.Rh.	0.9	41	31	25
8 J.deL.	0.4	84	66	21
9 D.E.	0.1	71	76	−7
10 R.T.	0.6	84	69	22
11 J.C.	0.2	21	23	−9
12 M.T.	0.2	21	12	43
13 S.Mc.	0.1	46	33	28
14a K.H.	0.2	31	28	10
14b K.H.	0.4	48	42	13
Mean	0.56			Mean 18.3

which accompany guanethidine administration.

The improved airway conductance values indicate that arginine does not irritate the airway. Mean arterial PO_2 approached the normal range for Denver, Colorado (67 to 75 mm Hg), probably as a result of improvement in ventilation and perfusion of the lung. Data obtained from rats given UC14 arginine indicated that 2 to 5% of arginine placed in the stomach appeared in the tracheal and bronchial fluids within an hour. Thus oral administration of arginine to patients with pulmonary disease may prove to be helpful in retarding the formation of mucous plugs *in situ*. We consider arginine to be a valuable addition to other forms of supportive therapy with prophylactic potential to minimize long term lung damage. No side effects have been noted over a period of 3 years. However, the risk of encountering a patient who has an adverse reaction to arginine administration must be borne in mind.

Part 2: Fat Absorption Studies

Increased intestinal absorptive ability in patients with severe pulmonary disease could be a result of improved pulmonary function. For this reason, patients with negligible pulmonary disease were selected for the gastrointestinal aspect of the study. Since bicarbonate protects pancreatic lipase from inactivation by hydrochloric acid,[9] the buffering action of arginine may have aided in stabilizing endogenous pancreatic lipase. It is known that oral bicarbonate administration is effective in improving absorption in patients with pancreatic exocrine insufficiency;[10] however, in our experience the use of an equivalent amount of arginine in this study decreased the fecal fat to a greater extent. This finding would suggest that additional properties of arginine such as its detergency and calcium-binding also contribute to increased fat absorption. Preliminary data suggests that mixed micelle formation, which is known to be of critical importance in the intraluminal phase of fat digestion, was enhanced by the *in vitro* addition of arginine to bile from three patients with cystic fibrosis. Patient 10 experienced a 22% decrease in fecal fat when given arginine in spite of an ileal resection which could have led to a state of bile salt deficiency. While the weight gain was well correlated to the decrease in fecal fat excretion, it is possible that stimulation of growth hormone and insulin by arginine may have played a part. All patients gained weight and in most cases this was the only significant increase in the previous 12 months. Preliminary data in three subjects with cystic fibrosis indicates that oral arginine acutely stimulated the secretion of both growth hormone and insulin.[11] However, studies in which serum samples were obtained at hourly intervals over a 24 hour period before and 1 month after the initiation of oral arginine did not demonstrate any change in the circadian serum pattern of these hormones. Acceptable agreement was seen in the decrease of fecal fat excretion both in the presence and absence of Cotazym administration in one patient (Table IV, 14a and 14b). Only one patient (12) was brought into the normal range of fat excretion. Three patients with mild steatorrhea (5, 11, 14a) did not increase their fat absorption but their abdominal pain was relieved. The relief of abdominal pain in an appreciable number of patients has also been reported using N-acetylcysteine[12] but its effect on steatorrhea has not been determined. Arginine, unlike N-acetylcysteine is probably not effective in breaking disulfide linkages which can contribute to the viscosity of mucus. However, arginine appears to be just as effective in the relief of abdominal pain and was more palatable to our patients. It remains to be seen whether the long-term oral administration of arginine will have a significant effect on the pathophysiology of mucoviscidosis. The patients also need to be observed for signs of calcium or other metal ion deficiencies which could result from the continued use of arginine. These studies are in progress.

SUMMARY

A total of 22 patients with cystic fibrosis were treated with buffered L-arginine given either as a mist to patients with pulmonary disease, or orally to those with predominantly gastrointestinal symptomatology. Arginine was selected because of its low toxicity, its ability to break hydrogen bonds, bind metal ions, and act as a detergent. The use of arginine was accompanied by significant improvements in vital capacity, thoracic gas volume, specific conductance, arterial Po_2, and intestinal fat absorption. The relief of abdominal pain and the lack of side effects indicated that L-arginine may be useful in the management of patients with cystic fibrosis. The complex physicochemical and pharmacological modes of action of L-arginine and its long-term effects warrant further clarification.

REFERENCES

1. DiSant', Agnese, P. A., and Talamo, R. C.: Pathogenesis and physiopathology of cystic fibrosis of the pancreas. N. Eng. J. Med., 227:1287, 1967.
2. Chernick, W. S., Barbero, G. J., and Perkins, F. M.: Studies on submaxillary saliva in cystic fibrosis. J. Pediat., 59:890, 1961.
3. Dubois, A. B., Botelho, S. Y., and Comroe, J. H., Jr.: A new method for measuring airway resistance in man using a body plethysmograph: Values in normal subjects and in patients with respiratory disease. J. Clin. Invest., 35:327, 1956.
4. Dubois, A. B., Botelho, S. Y., Bedell, G. N., Marshall, R., Comroe, J. H., Jr.,: A rapid plethysmographic method for measuring thoracic gas volume. J. Clin. Invest., 35:322, 1956.
5. Jensen, K. G.: Meconium-ileus equivalent in a 15 year old patient with mucoviscidosis. Acta Paediat. (Stockholm), 51:344, 1962.
6. Van de Kamer, J. H., Ten Bokkel Huinink, H., and Weijers, H. A.: Rapid method for determination of fat in feces. J. Biol. Chem., 177:347, 1949.
7. Gross, J., and Kirk, D.: Heat precipitation of collagen from neutral salt solutions: Some regulating factors. J. Biol. Chem., 233:355, 1958.
8. Chernick, W. S., Barbero, G. J., and Perkins, F. M.: Reversal of submaxillary salivary alterations in cystic fibrosis by guanethidine. In Rossi, E., and Stoll, E., ed.: Modern Problems in Pediatrics, Vol. 10. Switzerland: Karger, pp. 125–134, 1967.
9. Veeger, W., Abils, J., Hellemans, N., and Niewey, H. O.: Effect of sodium bicarbonate

and pancreatin on the absorption of Vitamin B_{12} and fat in pancreatic insuffiency. New Engl. J. Med. 267:134, 1962.

10. Davenport, H. W.: Physiology of the Digestive Tract, ed. 2. Chicago: Year Book Medical Publishers, Inc., pp. 130–140, 1966.

11. Gotlin, R. W., Solomons, C. C., and Cotton, E.: The influence of oral arginine on the plasma levels of insulin and growth hormone in subjects with cystic fibrosis. In preparation.

12. Gracey, M., Burke, V., and Anderson, C. M.: Treatment of abdominal pain in cystic fibrosis by oral administration of N-acetylcysteine. Arch. Dis. Child., 44:404, 1969.

13. Shwachman, H., and Kulczycki, L. L.: Long-term study of 105 patients with cystic fibrosis. Amer. J. Dis. Child., 96:6, 1958.

144

Carbenicillin in patients with cystic fibrosis: Clinical pharmacology and therapeutic evaluation

Nancy N. Huang, M.D., E. Joan Hiller, M.B., M.R.C.P.,
Carlos M. Macri, M.D., Marie Capitanio, M.D., and Kenneth R. Cundy, Ph.D.

CARBENICILLIN (carboxybenzylpenicillin), a new semisynthetic penicillin, has

Supported in part by a research grant from Charles Pfizer and Company, Inc., by Grant No. FR75 of the National Institutes of Health, by a center grant of the National Cystic Fibrosis Research Foundation, and by the Greater Delaware Valley Regional Medical Program.

only a slightly different side chain from ampicillin (amino-benzylpenicillin).[1] It is the first drug that is moderately active against *P. aeruginosa* and can be administered parenterally in large doses for prolonged periods without adverse effect. These advantages prompted us to study its clinical pharmacology and therapeutic effect on patients

145

with cystic fibrosis who had chronic pulmonary infections.

MATERIALS AND METHODS

In vitro susceptibility. All of the bacterial pathogens isolated from patients with cystic fibrosis before, during, and after treatment were tested for their susceptibility to carbenicillin and other antibiotic agents by the disc method.[2] A selected number of these organisms were also tested by the standard tube dilution method. Both minimal inhibitory concentration and minimal bactericidal concentration of carbenicillin were determined for a small number of strains of *P. aeruginosa,* Proteus spp., and Escherichia spp.

Combinations of carbenicillin with colistin and/or gentamicin were tested for synergy against carbenicillin-resistant strains of *P. aeruginosa.*[3] In these tests, stepwise dilutions of single antibiotics and of various combinations of 2 antibiotics were set up. Inocula of 10^6 organisms per milliliter of an overnight culture were then added to the broth containing antibiotic and incubated for 18 hours. The minimal inhibitory concentrations of the individual antibiotics and of combined antibiotics were determined and compared.

Sera. Serum samples were obtained from 5 patients for assay of carbenicillin before and at $\frac{1}{2}$, 2, 4, and 6 hour intervals following a single intravenous dose of carbenicillin. Three patients received oral probenecid before carbenicillin was given. Random samples were obtained from 29 patients during the therapeutic trial of carbenicillin with concurrent administration of probenecid. Paired serum and bronchial secretions were obtained from 8 patients at intervals of 1 to 2 hours following an intravenous dose of carbenicillin.

Renal excretion. Renal excretion was measured in 2 children following a single dose of 100 mg. per kilogram of carbenicillin given intravenously without probenecid for a period of 4 hours. Urine was collected for carbenicillin assay from 3 patients following single and repeated aerosol treatments with carbenicillin.

Standard agar-diffusion technique, using a sensitive strain of *Pseudomonas aeruginosa*

10490 as the testing organism, was employed for assay of carbenicillin in serum, urine, and bronchial secretions. (All assays were performed by the Charles Pfizer Medical Research Laboratories.)

Therapeutic evaluation. Carbenicillin was administered by the intravenous route to 54 children with cystic fibrosis during acute exacerbations of chronic pulmonary infections having *P. aeruginosa* as the predominant pathogen in throat cultures. Twenty-nine patients received a single course of treatment and 25 other patients received multiple courses for a total of 85 therapeutic trials. Each course of therapy lasted for 7 to 30 days with an average duration of 14 days. The daily dose ranged from 150 to 500 mg. per kilogram divided into 5 doses. Each dose of the antibiotic was added to a Buratrol chamber containing 20 to 30 ml. of 5 per cent glucose in 0.05M sodium chloride solution; the total volume was given intravenously in a period of 10 to 15 minutes. If such a dose were to be administered undiluted and rapidly, it would invariably cause severe pain.

During the period of carbenicillin administration, all oral antibiotic agents taken prior to hospitalization were discontinued, but physical therapy, use of a mist tent, and aerosol therapy with mucolytic agents and bronchodilators were continued as before.

In the case of strains of *P. aeruginosa* not inhibited or killed by 500 μg per milliliter of carbenicillin, or found to be resistant by the disc method (less than 20 mm. zone around disc), a combination of carbenicillin with colistin or of carbenicillin with gentamicin was employed, depending upon the results of sensitivity tests. The daily doses of colistin and gentamicin were 5 mg. per kilogram given at 12 hour intervals by intramuscular injection or by slow intravenous drip. Colistin or gentamicin was used in combination with carbenicillin for only 10 days during any course of treatment.

Therapeutic efficacy was evaluated through changes in the general condition of the patient, frequency and severity of coughing, sleeping respiratory rate, temperature, physical findings, weight gain, roentgenologic appearance of the chest, pulmonary function tests, and bacteriologic studies. Thirty-seven of the 54 patients treated had advanced disease. All patients had increased respiratory rate, moist rales and harsh breath sounds in the chest, and parenchymal infiltrations on chest roentgenograms prior to the administration of carbenicillin. It was therefore seldom difficult to determine whether the patients improved with therapy; it was extremely unusual, however, to achieve improvement in all clinical parameters.

Hemoglobin, white blood cell counts, differential cell counts, and platelet counts were obtained frequently during the course of therapy. Blood urea nitrogen and serum glutamic oxaloacetic transaminase were determined before and at the end of the course of therapy in most of the children studied.

RESULTS

In vitro susceptibility. Table I shows the susceptibility pattern of coagulase-positive *Staphylococcus aureus* to 7 antibiotic agents by the tube dilution method. Carbenicillin was moderately active against *S. aureus*. The majority of strains tested were susceptible to 6.25 μg per milliliter or less of carbenicillin. Methicillin and cephaloridine were very active against the strains tested. Twenty-five per cent of the strains tested were very sensitive to penicillin G; the rest were resistant. Nearly 40 per cent of the strains were sensitive to ampicillin; about 60 per cent of the strains tested were inhibited by 6.25 μg per milliliter of chloramphenicol. Most strains were resistant to tetracycline.

The susceptibility pattern of *P. aeruginosa* to 6 antibiotic agents is summarized in Table II; 40 per cent of the strains tested were inhibited by 62.5 μg per milliliter or less of carbenicillin. Most of the strains tested were highly susceptible to colistin and gentamicin. The inhibitory concentrations of Kanamycin, chloramphenicol, and tetracycline against *P. aeruginosa* were of a similar order.

No significant difference has been found in the susceptibility pattern of rough and mucoid strains of *P. aeruginosa* to the antibiotic agents tested. In a small number of selected strains tested, the mucoid variety was more sensitive than the rough kind.

Ninety-nine strains of *P. aeruginosa* were also tested for both minimal inhibitory concentration and minimal bactericidal concentration of carbenicillin. The results (Fig. 1) showed that 61 of 99 strains were killed by 250 μg per milliliter or less of carbenicillin.

Carbenicillin is highly effective against Proteus spp. and selected strains of Escherichia spp., Enterobacter, Serratia, Herellea, and Mima polymorpha but ineffective against *Klebsiella pneumoniae*. Carbenicillin is both inhibitory as well as bactericidal against most of the susceptible strains of Escherichia spp., Serratia marcescens, and Proteus spp. (Figs. 2 and 3).

An attempt was made to correlate carbenicillin sensitivities of *P. aeruginosa, E. coli,* and Proteus spp. as determined by the disc and tube-dilution methods. There was a lack of precise correlation between the 2 methods. Roughly, if one obtained a zone of 30 mm. of inhibition or greater around a 100 μg

Table I. Susceptibility pattern of 37 *Staphylococcus aureus* strains to 7 antibiotic agents

Antibiotic agents	No. of strains inhibited by antibiotic agents									
	Concentration of antibiotic in micrograms per milliliter									
	< 0.095	0.195	0.39	0.78	1.56	3.12	6.25	12.5	25	50 or >
Carbenicillin	0	0	0	9	5	9	10	3	0	1
Methicillin	0	0	0	2	8	23	3	0	1	0
Cephaloridine	0	0	0	36	1	0	0	0	0	0
Penicillin G	9	0	0	0	0	0	1	3	7	17
Ampicillin	0	0	0	9	0	5	4	2	2	15
Chloramphenicol	0	0	0	0	1	17	7	6	0	6
Tetracycline	5	0	0	1	1	0	0	0	1	29

disc, the organism was inhibited by 62.5 μg per milliliter or less of carbenicillin. If the disc method showed a zone of 20 mm. or less of inhibition, the organism was resistant by the tube-dilution method.

Concentration of carbenicillin in serum and bronchial secretion. Serum concentrations of carbenicillin following single intravenous doses of 40 to 90 mg. per kilogram showed very transient high peak levels which dropped to 5 μg per milliliter at the end of 2 hours (Table III). The concurrent administration of probenecid prolonged the high level to 2 hours with a gradual drop over 4 hours. Random serum levels following multiple intravenous doses of 60 to 100 mg. per kilogram per dose with concurrent oral ad-

ministration of probenecid showed effective levels for ½ to 2 hours following each dose. The assay of bronchial secretions following intravenous administration of carbenicillin revealed that despite the high serum levels, only 2 of 8 bronchial samples had detectable concentrations of carbenicillin.

Renal excretion. The renal excretion of carbenicillin in 4 hours after intravenous administration of a single dose of 100 mg. per kilogram without probenecid amounted to 86 per cent of the dose given in one patient and 76 per cent in another patient; these values are similar to the excretion patterns of other penicillin preparations.

Urinary excretion following aerosol administration amounted to only one per cent

Table II. Susceptibility pattern of *Pseudomonas aeruginosa*

Antibiotic agents	No. of strains tested	No. of strains inhibited by antibiotic agents (μg/ml.)						
		1.9 or less	3.8-7.8	15.6-31.2	62.5	125	250	500 or greater
Carbenicillin	110	5	10	7	22	39	18	9
Colistin	35	26	3	2	4	0	0	0
Gentamicin	35	30	4	0	1	0	0	0
Kanamycin	40	0	2	0	38	0	0	0
Chloramphenicol	40	0	0	0	40	0	0	0
Tetracycline	40	0	6	14	20	0	0	0

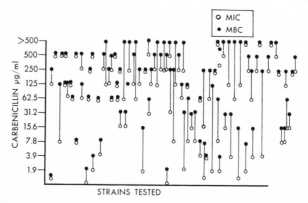

Fig. 1. Minimal inhibitory concentration (O) and minimal bactericidal concentration (●) of carbenicillin against 99 strains of *Pseudomonas aeruginosa*. The minimal inhibitory concentration and minimal bactericidal concentration of each strain are linked by a straight line. The ordinate depicts concentration of carbenicillin in micrograms per milliliter in twofold dilutions.

148

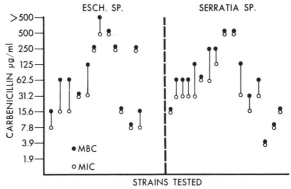

Fig. 2. Minimal inhibitory concentration (O) and minimal bactericidal concentration (●) of carbenicillin against 13 strains of Escherichia sp. and 16 strains of Serratia sp. The minimal inhibitory concentration and minimal bactericidal concentration of each strain are linked by a straight line. The ordinate depicts concentration of carbenicillin in micrograms per milliliter in twofold dilutons.

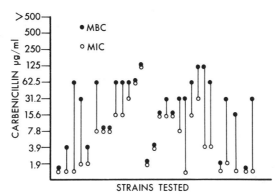

Fig. 3. Minimal inhibitory concentration (O) and minimal bactericidal concentration (●) of carbenicillin against 29 strains of Proteus sp. The minimal inhibitory concentration and minimal bactericidal concentration of each strain are linked by a straight line. The ordinate depicts concentration of carbenicillin in micrograms per milliliter in twofold dilutions.

of the dose nebulized, irrespective of the method used or the nature of the nebulizing solution in which carbenicillin was dissolved. No cumulative effect was found following multiple-dose aerosol therapy in 3 patients when given 4 times daily over a period of 7 days.

Therapeutic trials. The results of 7 therapeutic regimens were analyzed according to clinical and radiologic responses, as listed in Table IV. The clinical parameters were evaluated by one of the authors and the radiologic changes were evaluated by another, without knowledge of the therapeutic regimen employed in each case. Only 3 patients deteriorated during the course of carbenicillin therapy; all other patients either improved or showed no change with therapy. Those who improved are listed in Table IV. Those patients who had received several

Table III. Serum carbenicillin concentration following single intravenous dose with or without probenecid

Patient	Age (yr.)	Weight (Kg.)	Dose Total (Gm.)	Dose mg./Kg.	Serum concentration (µg/ml.) Pre-	½ hr.	2 hr.	4 hr.	6 hr.
R. C.	4	12	1.0	90	0	125	5	3.5	3.8
A. H.	14	25	1.0	40	0	157	5.5	3.5	3.8
D. H.	12	33	1.0*	30	0	153	85.7	14.0	3.8
W. S.	10½	30	3.0*	100	0	80	58.8	22.9	—
D. S.	14	35	3.0*	90	0	197	81.6	22.1	—

*With oral administration of probenecid.

Table IV. Therapeutic response of patients with cystic fibrosis to carbenicillin administration

Group	Therapeutic regimen	No. of patients	No. of patient days	Clinical response No. of patients improved	Rate of improvement per 2 wk. therapy* (%)	Radiologic response No. of patients improved	Rate of improvement per 2 wk. therapy* (%)
I	Carbenicillin intravenously 150 mg./Kg./day	11	123	3	34.1	2	22.8
II	Carbenicillin intravenously 200-250 mg./Kg./day	13	164	10	85.4	6	51.2
III	Carbenicillin intravenously 300-350 mg./Kg./day	14	165	8	67.9	10	84.8
IV	Carbenicillin intravenously 500 mg./Kg./day	20	266	13	68.4	10	52.6
V	Carbenicillin intravenously 500 mg./Kg./day + carbenicillin aerosol 500 mg. b.i.d.	7	96	4	58.3	3	43.8
VI	Carbenicillin intravenously 500 mg./Kg./day + colistin 5 mg./Kg./day intramuscularly or intravenously	13	199	10	70.3	6	42.2
VII	Carbenicillin intravenously 500 mg./Kg./day + gentamicin 5 mg./Kg./day intramuscularly or intravenously	7	114	5	61.4	3	36.8

*Rate of improvement for 2 week treatment period $= \dfrac{\text{Number of patients improved}}{\text{Total patient days of observation}} \times 14$ days.

different regimens were treated as different individuals in each group.

For those patients who were treated repeatedly with the same dosage regimen, the results of only one therapeutic course were analyzed. The response was summarized according to the rate of patient improvement over total number of patient days observed. Since the average duration of therapy was 14 days, the rate of patient improvement for 2 weeks of treatment was calculated for each group. In group I, only 34 per cent of patients improved clinically and 23 per cent improved radiologically during 2 weeks of

Table V. Bacterial pathogens isolated before and at the end of carbenicillin administration

Pathogen	Pre-treatment positive cultures	End-treatment positive cultures
Pseudomonas aeruginosa	85	57
Staphylococcus aureus	52	35
Proteus species	17	11
Escherichia coli	27	29
Klebsiella pneumoniae	8	35
Hemophilus influenzae	5	1
Serratia marcescens	2	2
Herellea	9	6
Mima polymorpha	0	4
Enterobacter aerogenes	2	4

treatment. For the remaining groups, clinical improvement ranged from 58 to 85 per cent, and radiologic improvement ranged from 37 to 85 per cent. The differences in the results obtained in the last 6 groups were not different from one another on statistical analysis. In our small series of patients treated, therefore, the over-all clinical and radiologic responses were not affected by the dose of carbenicillin administered so long as it was higher than 150 mg. per kilogram per day; nor was the response improved by the addition of aerosol inhalation. The addition of colistin or gentamicin also did not make any difference in our therapeutic results.

Most of the patients in groups 6 and 7 had advanced disease and had been treated repeatedly with carbenicillin. Some strains of *P. aeruginosa* isolated from those patients became highly resistant to carbenicillin; other patients had mixtures of both sensitive and resistant varieties. Synergistic effect between carbenicillin and colistin or between carbenicillin and gentamicin was demonstrated in some strains tested.

Bacteriologic responses were not different in the groups studied. The data are pooled and listed in Table V. The striking change in the end-treatment flora of these patients was the marked increase in isolations of *Klebsiella pneumoniae* which was uniformly resistant to carbenicillin.

SIDE EFFECTS

No instance of a hematologic disorder, renal toxicity, skin rash, or fever has been observed in the clinical trials of carbenicillin. An elevation of serum glutamic oxaloacetic transaminase activity in the post-treatment phase was found, however, in 32 of 82 therapeutic trials. The range of pretreatment levels of serum glutamic oxaloacetic transaminase was from 5 to 65 units with a median of 38; end-treatment levels were from 6 to 267 units with a median of 70 units.

DISCUSSION

All of the patients studied had high serum antibody titers to Pseudomonas antigen[4]; this observation supports the conclusion that *P. aeruginosa* plays an important role in the chronic pulmonary infections of these patients. Our results showed that carbenicillin is moderately active against *P. aeruginosa* and very active against selective strains of Proteus spp., Escherichia spp., Enterobacter aerogenes, and other gram-negative organisms. It is also fairly effective against coagulase-positive staphylococci.

Most of the patients treated with carbenicillin experienced a favorable clinical response in the form of reduction of cough, lowering of temperature, increase in appetite, and improvement in general condition. It usually took much longer for physical findings and roentgenologic manifestations to show improvement. The therapeutic effect of carbenicillin was impressive in some of the patients treated, but the improvement was of transient nature in those with advanced disease.

Despite clinical improvement in more than 50 per cent of patients treated with high doses of carbenicillin, it was extremely difficult to eradicate *P. aeruginosa* from the respiratory flora. The administration of carbenicillin by aerosol in combination with its intravenous administration in a small number of patients did not result in greater clinical improvement, nor did it prove to be beneficial from the standpoint of roentgenologic or bacteriologic findings.

The fact that carbenicillin must be administered intravenously is a definite disadvantage. It is apparent that this type of therapy cannot be carried out for prolonged periods of time. Patients with advanced disease, therefore, were treated with repeated courses of 2 to 3 weeks' duration.

The finding of strains of *P. aeruginosa* resistant to carbenicillin raises great concern in the prospective role of carbenicillin in the treatment of patients with cystic fibrosis. It is important to determine whether combined therapy with gentamicin or colistin will prevent the development of resistant strains in the future.

No significant toxicity to carbenicillin has been encountered, in particular no evidence of renal, hematologic or neurologic side effects have been observed. Eosinophilia, as reported by Boxerbaum,[5] was not detected in our patients. Transient elevations of serum glutamic oxaloacetic transaminase activity occurred in 40 per cent of our patients and was accompanied by a rise of serum glutamic pyruvate transaminase in a small number of them, none had increases in concentration of bilirubin or other changes in liver function tests.

The authors are grateful to Anita Brody, B.S., A.S.C.P., and Nancy Haney, B.S., A.S.C.P., for technical assistance, to Shirley Braverman, M.S., for statistical analysis, to Yung Yong, B.S., for art work, to Maurice Goldberg, our pharmacist, for invaluable assistance in keeping records of our drug supply and preparing carbenicillin for clinical use, to Helen Reck, R.N., and Linda Wassum, R.N., for clinical assistance, to all resident and nursing staff for patient care, and to Anthony Knirsch, M.D., for generously supplying carbenicillin.

REFERENCES

1. Acred, P., Brown, D. M., Knudson, E. T., Robinson, G. N., and Sutherland, R.: New semi-synthetic penicillin active against Pseudomonas pyocyanea, Nature 215: 25, 1967.
2. Bauer, A. W., Kirby, W. M. M., Sherris, J. C., and Turck, M.: Antibiotic susceptibility testing by a standardized single disc method, Amer. J. Clin. Path. 45: 493, 1966.
3. Garrod, L. P., and O'Grady, F.: Antibiotic and chemotherapy, Baltimore, 1968, The Williams & Wilkins Company, p. 448.
4. Huang, N. N., Cundy, K., Tongudai, S., and Cuasay, L.: Serum antibody titer to pseudomonas of patients with cystic fibrosis, Cystic Fibrosis Club, 11th Annual Meeting 1970, Abstract, p. 19.
5. Boxerbaum, B., Doershuk, C. F., Pittman, S., and Mathews, L. W.: Efficacy and tolerance of carbenicillin in patients with cystic fibrosis, Antimicrob. Agents Chemother. 1968, p. 292.

152

FUSIDIC ACID AND LINCOMYCIN THERAPY IN STAPHYLOCOCCAL INFECTIONS IN CYSTIC FIBROSIS

GORDON L. T. WRIGHT   JAMES HARPER

Summary An investigation was done in eighteen patients with cystic fibrosis who had had pulmonary infection with *Staphylococcus aureus* for known durations of one month to nine years, with the dual objectives of eliminating this infection and preventing reinfection. Fusidic acid was used in conjunction with lincomycin, chloramphenicol, cloxacillin, phenoxymethylpenicillin, and novobiocin. Staphylococci were eliminated in sixteen patients, fifteen when fusidic acid was combined with lincomycin and two (one reinfection) when combined with novobiocin. Combinations with chloramphenicol and the penicillins were unsuccessful. In four patients staphylococci became resistant to lincomycin, and in two of these the staphylococci also became resistant to fusidic acid. Two patients developed bronchopneumonia due to *Pseudomonas æruginosa* during fusidic acid and lincomycin therapy, soon after the sputa became clear of staphylococci. Gastrointestinal complications were not seen. After twenty successful treatments, prophylaxis was tried with tetracycline, aerosol neomycin, or lincomycin. Fifteen of the sixteen patients given continuous prophylactic lincomycin still had negative sputa after periods from five to nineteen months. The single reinfection was by an organism of a different phage type. Prophylaxis with tetracycline or aerosol neomycin was unsuccessful.

153

Introduction

PULMONARY complications and infections are the predominant factors in the long-term prognosis for patients with cystic fibrosis. *Staphylococcus aureus* has been consistently found in a large proportion of cystic-fibrosis patients, usually accompanied by gram-negative organisms, especially *Pseudomonas æruginosa*. We find staphylococci in the sputum of 80% of patients, and others have reported frequencies of 95% (18/19) [1] and 70% (9/13).[2] Patterson et al.[3] found staphylococci in the bronchial washings of 17 of 25 patients. Mitchell et al.[4] showed that patients with chronic lung disease are liable to acquire staphylococcal lung infections if they are kept in hospital more than seven days, and they advised against admission whenever possible.

A history of clinical deterioration often dates back to a pulmonary staphylococcal infection; once established, such infections are very difficult to eradicate, and even if this is achieved reinfection usually occurs within a short period. We have been using mucolytic agents and aerosols combined with postural drainage preceded by bronchodilatation for some years but have been disappointed at the lack of real improvement in the smaller children with staphylococcal pulmonary infection.

Saggers and Lawson [5] have suggested that antibiotics which diffuse well into mucus might be helpful in the management of cystic fibrosis. Using hog mucin to simulate the in-vivo situation, they investigated a series of antibiotics and found that (apart from the sulphonamides), erythromycin, lincomycin, and fusidic acid penetrated the mucus most extensively.

Since many of our patients had already received erythromycin, we decided to investigate the efficacy of fusidic acid in combination with another antibiotic, usually lincomycin, in eradicating staphylococcal infection from the lungs. Fusidic acid was used with another antibiotic to forestall, if possible, the emergence of resistant organisms.[6]

Once the infection had been eradicated, treatment was continued prophylactically with a single antibiotic, usually lincomycin.

Patients and Methods

Patients

18 children aged from eighteen months to fifteen years (9 males and 9 females) attended the cystic-fibrosis research clinic of the University of Queensland for investigation and treatment. In all, the diagnosis of cystic fibrosis was established both by clinical history and sweat electrolytes. The known duration of staphylococcal infection ranged from one month to nine years (table I). The duration was dated from the first positive culture recorded, but since in many patients no such record was available before referral to this clinic, the duration was almost certainly very much longer than the stated time in most patients. All had received treatment with penicillin, tetracycline, erythromycin, and often with chloramphenicol. There had often been some clinical benefit but no influence on the persistence of the infection. During this investigation, 18 patients had a total of thirty treatments (tables I and II).

Investigations

In all patients the presence of *Staph. aureus* was demonstrated by culture of sputum or cough swabs. Specimens were inoculated on blood-agar plates and colonies of staphylococci were tested for coagulase production. Coagulase-positive staphylococci were phage-typed and were tested for sensitivity to antibiotics by the disc diffusion method. The strengths of discs used were (μg.): gentamicin 10, lincomycin 2, fucidin 10, and novobiocin 30. Evans ' Sentest H.P.' tablets were used for the other antibiotic discs.

Nasal swabs were also taken from the patients and, where possible, from the other members of the household. Almost all patients with staphylococci in the sputum (or cough swab) had one or more members of the household with positive nasal swabs, but not always of the same phage type.

When possible, sputum cultures were done daily during treatment. During prophylaxis, sputum cultures were done on each visit to the clinic, usually weekly for the first month, then monthly for two or three months, then according to the patient's clinical condition. Weekly follow-up was not possible in some patients living long distances from Brisbane but in each case subsequent follow-up was adequate.

Where the child was old enough to cooperate, pulmonary function was assessed by measurement of the peak expiratory flow-rate, forced expiratory volumes in 0·5 and 1 second, and the forced vital capacity.

Therapeutic Management

Fusidic acid was used in all patients, always combined with another antibiotic and given in divided doses every six hours. The dosage of fusidic acid was 800 mg. daily for the

155

TABLE I—TREATMENT AND PROPHYLAXIS IN 18 PATIENTS (THIRTY TREATMENTS)

Patient	Sex	Age (yr.)	Treatment				Prophylaxis		
			Known duration of infection (yr.)	Antibiotic with fusidic acid	Duration of treatment (days)	Result	Antibiotic	Duration	Result
A	M	1½	3/12	Lin.	14	Success	Lin.	8 mo.	Clear
B	M	4	3/12	Lin.	14	Success	Lin.	8 mo.	Clear
C	F	22/12	3/12	Lin.	14	Success	Lin.	13 mo.	Clear
D	F	20/12	1/12	Lin.	8	Success	Lin.	8 mo.	Clear
E	M	3	3	Lin. & Amp. Nov.	13	Failure	..	..	..
E	M	3	..		8	Failure			..
F	M	3	9/12	Lin.	21	Success	Aer., Neo.	18 days	Relapse
F	M	4	7/12	Lin.	13	Success	Lin.	11 mo.	Clear
G	F	4	2	Lin.	21	Success	Aer. Neo.	18 days	Relapse
G	F	5	7/12	Lin.	13	Success	Lin.	11 mo.	Clear
							Ery.	9 mo.	Clear
H	F	4	..	Lin.	19	Success	Lin.	12 mo.	Clear
I	F	10	5	Lin.	19	Doubtful	Ery.	18 days	Relapse
I	F	10	..	Chlor.	13	Failure	Chlor. & Lin.	6 wk.	Relapse
I	F	11	..	Nov.	21	Success	Lin.	5 mo.	Clear

J	M	6	3	Lin.	10	Success	Lin. & Amp.	10 mo.	Clear
K	M	8	4	Lin.	14	Failure	..	..	..
K	M	8	..	Nov.	14	Failure	..	..	..
L	M	8	2¹/₂	Pen V	19	Failure	..	..	Clear
L	M	8	..	Lin.	18	Success	Lin.	19 mo.	Clear
M	M	7	4	Lin.	12	Success	Lin.	5 mo.	Clear (died)
N	M	7	6	Pen V.	26 ⎫	Failure	..	..	..
N	M	7	..	Clox.	18 ⎬ 58	Failure	..	..	Relapse
N	M	8	..	Lin.	14 ⎭	Success	Aer. Neo.	17 days	..
N	M	8	..	Chlor.	16	Failure	..	..	..
N	M	8	..	Lin.	16	Success	Lin.	5 mo.	Clear
O	F	13	9	Lin.	20	Success	Lin.	17 mo.	Clear
P	F	14	3/12	Lin.	14	Success	Lin.	2 mo.	Relapse
P	F	14	..	Nov.	20	Success	Lin.	5 mo.	Clear
Q	F	14	2	Lin.	21	Success	Lin.	16 mo.	Clear
R	F	15	9	Lin.	21	Success	Tetra.	2 mo.	Relapse

(Bracketed patients are siblings). Lin. = lincomycin; Chlor. = chloramphenicol; Pen V. = phenoxymethylpenicillin; Clox. = cloxacillin; Amp. = ampicillin; Tetra. = tetracycline; Ery. = erythromycin; Neo. = neomycin; Nov. = novobiocin. Duration of prophylaxis means time to recurrence, or time after which the sputa are still negative.

younger children and 1000 mg. daily for the older patients
(23–50 mg. per kg.); for lincomycin, phenoxymethylpenicillin, and cloxacillin, 1000 mg. daily (23–50 mg. per
kg.); for chloramphenicol, 750 mg. daily (34–40 mg. per
kg.); and for novobiocin, 500 mg. or 1000 mg. daily
(23–33 mg. per kg.).

Details of duration of infection, the antibiotic used, the
duration of treatment, and the results are shown in table I,
and the results summarised in table II. In all patients
treated, the staphylococci were reported to be sensitive to
the antibiotics used, except for 2 patients treated with penicillin. Penicillin was used in these cases combined with
fusidic acid since the two antibotics are said to act syner-
gistically in vitro against penicillinase-producing staphylococci.[7]

Treatment was continued until negative sputa had been
obtained for one week, which, with the time taken for culture, usually meant nine days from the first negative sputum.
Routine general measures using postural drainage and
mucolytic agents were continued; where patients had been
having aerosols of neomycin or of kanamycin with polymyxin, these were continued.

Results

TREATMENT

The combination of fusidic acid and lincomycin
proved highly successful; staphylococci were elimin-

TABLE II—RESULTS OF TREATMENT WITH FUSIDIC ACID COMBINED
WITH OTHER ANTIBIOTICS IN 18 PATIENTS AND PROPHYLAXIS AFTER
TWENTY SUCCESSFUL TREATMENTS

Regimen	Patients	Treat-ments	Success	Failure	Doubtful
Fusidic acid with:					
Lincomycin ..	18	21	18	2	1
Chloramphenicol	2	2	0	2	0
Penicillin V ..	2	2	0	2	0
Cloxacillin ..	1	1	0	1	0
Novobiocin ..	4	4	2	2	0
Total	..	30	20	9	1
Prophylaxis after 20 successful treatments:					
Lincomycin ..	16	0	15	1	0
Erythromycin ..	1	0	1	0	0
Tetracycline ..	1	0	0	1	0
Aerosol neomycin	3	0	0	3	0
Total ..	21*	0	16	5	0

* 1 patient had prophylaxis first by erythromycin then by lincomycin
following the one successful treatment.

158

ated in eighteen of twenty-one treatments, two were unsuccessful and the other doubtful. In terms of patients, this combination was used in 18 and was successful in 15. Table II shows that combinations of fusidic acid with chloramphenicol, phenoxymethylpenicillin, and cloxacillin were unsuccessful. In the 4 patients who received four treatments with fusidic acid and novobiocin, the combination was successful in 2 and failed in 2. Staphylococcal resistance to fusidic acid developed in the 2 patients who did not respond to fusidic acid with lincomycin or novobiocin. A combination of ' Fucidin ' (sodium salt of fusidic acid) and novobiocin was used in 3 patients whose staphylococci had become resistant to lincomycin (E, I, K), and also in patient P who acquired a lincomycin-resistant strain.

Complications of Treatment

Gastrointestinal complications.—There were hardly any gastrointestinal complications from fusidic acid and lincomycin in these patients despite the relatively high doses used.

Bronchopneumonia.—2 patients, J and R, developed a bronchopneumonia while having therapy with fusidic acid and lincomycin but after the sputum was reported negative for staphylococci. This condition was associated in each case with a leucoctyosis of about 35,000 per c.mm., a heavy growth of *Ps. æruginosa* in the sputum, and an asthmatic type of expiratory respiratory distress with gross overinflation of the lungs. Patient J responded to treatment with gentamicin parentally and chloramphenicol, and patient R responded to colistin.

Novobiocin toxicity.—Novobiocin was associated with toxicity in 3 of 4 patients treated. P (aged fifteen years) became jaundiced, but this cleared rapidly when novobiocin was withdrawn; E (aged three and a half years) developed urticarial lesions which disappeared when novobiocin was stopped and reappeared when recommenced; and K (aged eight years) complained of abdominal pain.

PROPHYLACTIC MANAGEMENT

Fusidic acid was not used prophylactically because we wished to prevent the emergence of resistant organisms as much as possible, and preferred to keep

TABLE III—EMERGENCE OF RESISTANT STAPHYLOCOCCI

Patient	Date	Phage type	Treatment (mg./kg./day)	Duration (days)	Sensitivity Fuc.	Sensitivity Lin.	Prophylaxis (mg./kg./day)	Duration	Sensitivity Fuc.	Sensitivity Lin.
E	Feb. 14, 1969	53/54/85	Fuc. 57 Lin. 72 Amp. 36	13	S	S	{ Lin. 30 Amp. 30	14 days	S	R
	April 20, 1969	53/54/85	Fuc. 50 Nov. 50	8	R	R	:	:	:	:
K	Oct. 1, 1968	52/80/81	Fuc. 40 Lin. 40	10 + 4	R	S	:	:	:	:
	April 22, 1969	52/80/81	Fuc. 40 Lin. 40	4	R	R	:	:	:	:
	May 15, 1969	52/80/81	Fuc. 40 Nov. 40	14	R	R	:	:	:	:
I	Nov. 9, 1967	52/52A/80	Fuc. 48 Lin. 48	19	Nil	Nil	Ery. 36	18 days	S	S
	Feb. 6, 1968	52/52A/80	Fuc. 48 Chlor. 36	13	Nil	Nil	{ Lin. 24 Chlor. 36	28 days	Nil	Nil
	Feb. 21, 1969	52/52A/80	Fuc. 48 Nov. 48	21	Nil	Nil	{ Lin. 24 Amp. 36	14 days 5 mo.	S Nil	R Nil
N	July 25, 1967	52/52A/80	Fuc. 53 Pen V. 53 Fuc. 53 Clox. 53	26 18 } 58	S S	S S	:	:	:	:
	Jan. 30, 1968	52/52A/80	Fuc. 53 Lin. 53 Fuc. 53 Lin. 53	14 10 } 26	Nil S	Nil R	Aer. 300 mg. Neo.	18 days	S	S
	Jan. 28, 1969	52/52A/80	Fuc. 53 Chlor. 40 Fuc. 53 Lin. 53	16 16	Nil Nil	Nil Nil	Chlor. 40 Lin. 40	10 days 5 mo.	S Nil	R Nil

Sensitivity = sensitivity at end of treatment or prophylaxis.
Duration = duration of treatment or duration of prophylaxis until resistant organisms found.
Nil = no staphylococci isolated.

it in reserve against staphylococci which might develop resistance to other antibiotics. Lincomycin at a dosage of 100–250 mg. twice daily, according to the age of the patient, was continued in those patients treated therapeutically with fusidic acid and lincomycin. Erythromycin was given to 1 patient at a dosage of 250 mg. twice daily for nine months. Prophylaxis was then continued with lincomycin.

Results

Details of the time of reappearance of staphylococci or duration of freedom to date are shown in table I, and the prophylactic management is summarised in table II. In 15 of the 16 patients treated prophylactically with lincomycin after successful therapy with fusidic acid and lincomycin, the sputum has remained free of staphylococci for periods ranging from five to nineteen months. The only failure (patient P) was due to a reinfection after two months with a lincomycin-resistant staphylococcus of a different phage type, which was subsequently eliminated by a combination of fusidic acid and novobiocin. The patient (Q) was given prophylactic erythromycin followed by lincomycin and remained clear during both courses. Staphylococci reappeared within two months in one patient aged 15 years treated prophylactically with tetracycline 750 mg. daily. There was also a recurrence in seven to eighteen days in 3 patients given neomycin aerosol, 2 of whom were treated simultaneously with an antibiotic cream containing neomycin and chlorhexidine to the nares.

Complications of Prophylaxis

The only complication noticed in the lincomycin prophylaxis was the tendency of gram-negative organisms to increase in the sputum, especially in those children who had much lung damage.

EMERGENCE OF RESISTANT STAPHYLOCOCCI

In four patients (E, K, I, and N) the staphylococci became resistant to lincomycin; in 2 of these (E and K) the organisms also acquired resistance to fusidic acid. Table III shows details of time relationships, phage types, dosage, and duration of treatment and prophylaxis, and development of resistance to lincomycin and fusidic acid.

161

Patient E was given lincomycin prophylaxis after treatment with lincomycin and fusidic acid for thirteen days. He was discharged for social reasons after several negative sputa but a specimen taken a day before discharge contained staphylococci sensitive to both antibiotics. Two weeks after discharge resistance to lincomycin was present. A few weeks later he was treated with fusidic acid and novobiocin but developed a toxic urticarial reaction within seven days. Resistance to both fusidic acid and lincomycin was found in all specimens examined subsequently.

Patient K ceased treatment with fusidic acid and lincomycin after ten days in October, 1968, through a misunderstanding. Five days later treatment was recommenced but ceased after another four days when resistance to fusidic acid was reported. This resistance seemed to disappear over the next few months and this treatment was repeated, but resistance to both fusidic acid and lincomycin was present within a few days. Sensitivity to fusidic acid was reported in several specimens over the next few weeks and he was treated with fusidic acid and novobiocin. Treatment was withdrawn at the end of two weeks because of abdominal pains and because the staphylococci were again resistant to both fusidic acid and lincomycin.

In *patient I* the staphylococci became resistant to lincomycin during prophylaxis with lincomycin. This followed treatment with fusidic acid and chloramphenicol and then prophylaxis for four weeks with lincomycin and chloramphenicol. The resistant organisms were subsequently eliminated with fusidic acid and novobiocin, and the sputum has remained clear for five months on lincomycin prophylaxis.

In *patient N* resistance to lincomycin did not develop until the second treatment with fusidic acid and lincomycin. This resistance disappeared over the next six months after which staphylococci were successfully eliminated by fusidic acid and lincomycin. The sputum was still clear after five months of lincomycin prophylaxis.

Patients E and K were the only patients in whom staphylococci were reported sensitive to lincomycin but resistant to erythromycin before treatment. In such patients treatment needs careful supervision and probably needs to be more prolonged; perhaps also the dosage of lincomycin should be increased to counter the well known cross resistance between these two antibiotics. Staphylococci appeared to develop resistance to lincomycin rather easily, especially if prophylactic doses were given without complete elimination of the infection.

Fusidic acid was never given alone and the development of resistance to this antibiotic when used with lincomycin or novobiocin was most disappointing.

Discussion

It is too early yet to assess what improvement can be expected from overcoming the staphylococcal infections but we have noticed that on the whole the younger children showed greater improvement. The first eight children in table I have shown considerable clinical progress (even E) as manifested by weight gain, decreased coughing, and increased activity and well-being. Potential improvement probably depends upon the extent of previous lung damage and this could explain the response of some of the older children. For example, patient Q (now aged fifteen) who had minimal lung changes now wins the 440-yard races at school, represents her school in cross-country races, and climbs mountains; patient P (aged fifteen) who radiologically had extensive patchy infiltration throughout the lungs but a reasonable vital capacity now wins the school swimming races. However, patients I and N, who have extensive bronchiectasis and a poor vital capacity have made little progress during the five months their sputa have remained free of staphylococci.

Patient M died from hepatic failure which was present before this therapy was commenced.

Perhaps the most satisfactory result was in patient L who had a persisting staphylococcal pulmonary infection after pneumonia two and a half years previously which left him with moderate lung damage. His second treatment (table I) was during admission for a right-sided spontaneous pneumothorax with a fully collapsed lung, and a heavy growth of *Staph. aureus* and *Ps. æruginosa* in the sputum. Sputa became negative for staphylococci nine days after commencing fusidic acid and lincomycin and after eighteen days he was given lincomycin prophylaxis 250 mg. twice daily. He had two further admissions for recurrences of the pneumothorax and a thoracotomy at which the leaking bullæ were oversewn. Despite his admission to hospital and the presence of staphylococci in the nasal swabs of his father and brother, his sputa have remained negative for the nineteen months he has been continuing with the lincomycin prophylaxis. He has pro-

163

gressed very well clinically (growth, games, swimming, school) but has had only a slight increase in pulmonary function. *Ps. æruginosa* have persisted in the sputum throughout.

Saggers and Lawson [5] and Lawson [8] showed in-vitro that fusidic acid, erythromycin, lincomycin, and novobiocin penetrated well through mucus, but that most of the other antibiotics did not. This investigation provides clinical evidence to support these in-vitro findings as shown by the efficacy of fusidic acid with lincomycin or novobiocin in our 18 patients.

No doubt erythromycin could be used with fusidic acid in suitable patients but most of these patients had already been treated with erythromycin.

Ker [9] and Penman [10] reported satisfactory results from combining fusidic acid with novobiocin. In our hands novobiocin has been too toxic to be viewed with favour but it has a role in the treatment of lincomycin-resistant staphylococcal infections.

Aerosol neomycin and the antibiotic cream were given on the principle that if the routes of access were blocked, reinfection should not happen. The failure of aerosol neomycin as a prophylactic agent throws grave doubt on its therapeutic value at least in the concentrations used (100 mg. each inhalation of 2 ml.).

Our failures with the fusidic acid and lincomycin combination seem to be the result of insufficient length of treatment in patients with long-standing infection. A few patients produced a positive sputum after several daily negatives, and we consider that treatment should be continued for at least three weeks and until the sputum has been clear of staphylococci for at least ten days.

The 2 patients with bronchopneumonia due to *Ps. æruginosa* were seriously ill and caused great concern since they had been reasonably well previously. Clinically, these cases resembled severe acute asthma, and the mothers of both were severe asthmatics. Bronchopneumonia developed about nine months after the start of this investigation, and after 7 or 8 children had been treated without any untoward effects, even though some of these had a heavy growth of this organism from their sputa. After this experience we proceeded much more cautiously when significant numbers of gram-negative organisms were found in the sputum and have taken measures to prevent undue ascendency of such infections.

Alternative methods of achieving the same results may be found, but we feel that with this combination of drugs we have found one satisfactory way to eradicate staphylococci from the lungs and to prevent their re-establishment. Our results have improved as we have gathered experience. We believe that the problems we encountered in Queensland are similar to those to be found in other places.

We would make the following suggestions to those who wish to embark upon this therapy:

(a) Supportive measures to remove mucus from the lungs are required: no antibiotic regimen will overcome the mechanical problem of airway obstruction by large quantities of viscid mucus nor deal with the excellent culture medium so provided.

(b) Good bacteriological supervision is needed both during treatment and prophylaxis.

(c) The staphylococci should be sensitive to both fusidic acid and lincomycin.

(d) Treatment with these antibiotics should be continued for at least three weeks, and at least until staphylococci have been absent from the sputum for ten days. It is not unusual in old-established infections to have a positive sputum several days after a series of negatives.

(e) Lincomycin is a narrow-spectrum antibiotic and does not cover the secondary invasion which often follows recurrent upper-respiratory-tract infection in these children. They may need in addition other antibiotics such as tetracycline, chloramphenicol, or ampicillin in the event of such infections. Where these are given, prophylactic lincomycin should not be suspended but continued as before.

(f) Where a heavy growth of gram-negative organisms is present before treatment, or where these are increasing during prophylaxis, another antibiotic is needed in addition to lincomycin and fusidic acid. We have been using ampicillin and/or aerosol gentamicin for this purpose.

Treatment with fusidic acid and lincomycin may be found useful in other staphylococcal infections with problems of accessibility similar to those of cystic fibrosis.

We thank Leo Pharmaceutical Products, Denmark (who supplied the fusidic acid through their Australian representatives, Ethnor Pty. Ltd.); Upjohn Pty. Ltd. who supplied the lincomycin; Miss Yvonne Battey of the Laboratory of Microbiology and Pathology, Brisbane, for the phage-typing; and the pædiatricians who allowed access to their patients. This work was done with the aid of a research grant from the Brisbane Children's Hospital Foundation.

REFERENCES

1. Feigelson, J., Pecau, Y. *Mod. Probl. Pædiat.* 1967, **10**, 214.
2. Haung, N. N., Kung-Tso, S. *J. Pediat.* 1963, **62**, 36.
3. Patterson P. R., Estilo, A.E., Stranahan, A. *Mod. Probl. Pædiat.* 1967, **10**, 315.
4. Mitchell, A. A. B., Dunn, R. I. S., Lees, T. S. *Lancet*, 1961, ii, 669.
5. Saggers, B. A., Lawson, D. *J. clin. Path.* 1966, **19**, 313.
6. Jensen, K., Lassen, H. C. A. *Q. Jl Med.* 1969, **38**, 91.
7. Barber, M., Waterworth, P. *Lancet*, 1962, i, 931.
8. Lawson, D. *Mod. Probl. Pædiat.* 1967, **10**, 332.
9. Ker, H. *Br. J. clin. Pract.* 1965, **19**, 227.
10. Penman, R. *Lancet*, 1962, ii, 1277.

The effect of isoproterenol on airway obstruction in cystic fibrosis

Elizabeth A. Featherby, M.B., M.R.C.P.(Lond.),

Tzong-Ruey Weng, M.D. and Henry Levison, M.D.

The pattern of ventilatory dysfunction showing increasing airway obstruction has been well documented in patients with cystic fibrosis.[1-3] Bronchodilator drugs have been recommended for use as part of the therapeutic regimen,[4] but convincing evidence of their effectiveness is lacking.[1-3, 5] In addition, in a study of the interrelationships of air flow, lung volume

and transpulmonary pressure in 13 patients with cystic fibrosis before and after the administration of racemic epinephrine, little change was found in the maximal flow rates and the pressures at which these were achieved, and by inference, little change in the mechanical properties of the lung.[6] This study was undertaken to assess the effectiveness of isoproterenol inhalation in relieving various degrees of airway obstruction in patients with cystic fibrosis of the pancreas.

Material and Methods

Forty-seven patients with cystic

From the Research Institute of The Hospital for Sick Children and the Department of Pediatrics, University of Toronto, Toronto, Ontario.
Supported by a grant from the Canadian Cystic Fibrosis Foundation.

fibrosis, 24 females and 23 males between the ages of 6 and 27 years and with heights ranging from 108 to 176 cm., were studied on 95 occasions to evaluate the bronchodilating effect of isoproterenol hydrochloride. The diagnosis of cystic fibrosis had been established by clinical criteria, sweat tests and radiological findings. Routine treatment (including prophylactic antibiotics, mist tent, physiotherapy and enzyme replacement) was not interrupted while the tests were made.

Initial spirometric measurements of the forced vital capacity (FVC), forced expiratory volume in one second ($FEV_{1.0}$), $FEV_{1.0}/FVC\%$, maximal mid-expiratory flow rate ($MMEF_{25\%-75\%}$) and maximal breathing capacity (MBC), were recorded on a 9-litre valveless spirometer.* Three recordings were made of each maneuver, and the greatest measurement was accepted and corrected to body temperature at saturated water vapour pressure (BTPS). In 27 of the 95 studies, measurements of the functional residual capacity (FRC_{He}) by the helium dilution technique* were also made, together with the thoracic gas volume (TGV) and airway resistance (R_{aw}) in a 510-litre body plethysmograph,* the last two in triplicate.[7-9] Measurements in normal children and young adults had already been made in our laboratory.[10]

Isoproterenol inhalation was withheld for at least four hours before the study was begun. The patient was then given 2.5 mg. isoproterenol hydrochloride by inhalation with a Bennett's nebulizer,* using compressed air at 7 litres per minute. Five minutes after completion of the inhalation, all spirometric measurements were repeated, together with the TGV and R_{aw} in those 27 studies in which they had been recorded initially.

We have previously shown that in asthmatic children the maximal effect from isoproterenol occurs from five to 15 minutes after the inhalation.[11]

Results

The results were assessed in two ways: (1) absolute values obtained before were compared to those obtained after bronchodilator administration, and (2) the values expressed as a percentage of our predicted normal values according to height[12] obtained before were compared to those obtained after bronchodilator administration. The changes due to treatment were analyzed using the paired data t-test.

The measurements were not expressed as a percentage of the initial values[13-15] because this method does not demonstrate the initial severity of the obstruction. For example, in one patient the MMEF of 0.25 litre per sec. increased to 0.70 litre per sec., 180% improvement over the initial value. Expressed as a percentage of the predicted normal value, however, this represents an improvement of 18% (from an original 10% to 28%).

---

*Warren E. Collins Inc., 220 Wood Road, Braintree, Mass. 02184.

Fig. 1 shows the initial $FEV_{1.0}$ values in relation to our normal data, according to height. Of the 95 studies performed, 73 showed

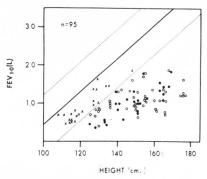

FIG. 1—Initial $FEV_{1.0}$ measurements, plotted against height, shown in relation to the regression line and 95% confidence limits for our normal data.

X — studies within the 95% confidence limits for the $FEV_{1.0}$
o — studies outside 95% confidence limits for the $FEV_{1.0}$
● — studies outside 95% confidence limits for the $FEV_{1.0}$ with additional FRC_{He}, TGV and R_{aw} measurements.

the initial $FEV_{1.0}$ to be outside and 22 within the 95% confidence limits for our normal data.

The initial MMEF measurements (Fig. 2) show a wider scatter than the $FEV_{1.0}$ values, but there is a wider scatter in our own normal MMEF measurements.

Fig. 3 demonstrates those 22 initial $FEV_{1.0}$ results within the 95% confidence limits, expressed as a percentage of our predicted normal values. It also shows the distribution of the MMEF values of the same group. Those 73 studies with the initial $FEV_{1.0}$ results outside the 95% confidence limits are expressed similarly in Fig. 4 and show a far greater shift to the left. In all studies the $FEV_{1.0}$ is higher than the MMEF, for this measurement includes the initial part of the flow volume curve

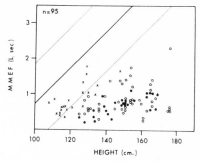

FIG. 2—Initial MMEF measurements plotted against height, shown in relation to the regression line and 95% confidence limits for our normal data.

X — studies within the 95% confidence limits for the $FEV_{1.0}$
o — studies outside 95% confidence limits for the $FEV_{1.0}$
● — studies outside 95% confidence limits for the $FEV_{1.0}$ with additional FRC_{He}, TGV and R_{aw} measurements.

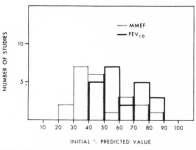

FIG. 3—Initial measurements (22 studies within the 95% confidence limits for the $FEV_{1.0}$) of the $FEV_{1.0}$ and MMEF expressed as percentages of the predicted normal values.

which is effort-dependent, whereas the MMEF maneuver is limited by the elastic recoil pressure of the lung, the frictional resistance of the small airways, and the cross-sectional area of large airways,[16] and is independent of effort.

The changes following isoproterenol administration on the 73 $FEV_{1.0}$ values outside and the 22 values inside the 95% confidence limits are analyzed separately, and

TABLE I
Effect of isoproterenol in 37 patients (73 studies) with cystic fibrosis

Measurement	Mean value I* (± S.D.) II**		Mean % predicted value I* (± S.D.) II**		P value
FVC (l.)	1.71 ± .59	1.83 ± .62	57.4 ±15.6	61.6 ±16.0	< .001
FEV$_{1.0}$ (l.)	1.06 ± .35	1.11 ± .38	40.7 ±11.3	42.9 ±13.0	< .02 > .01
MMEF (l./sec.)	0.79 ± .37	0.98 ± .46	25.8 ±12.2	31.9 ±13.6	< .001
MBC (l./min.)	59.8 ±18.8	65.5 ±19.2	63.2 ±13.9	69.3 ±13.6	< .001
FEV$_{1.0}$/VC%	60.5 ±13.9	58.5 ±11.7	—		< .05 > 0.01

*Before bronchodilator administration.
**After bronchodilator administration.

TABLE II
Mean changes in 22 studies, in which the initial FEV$_{1.0}$ was within the 95% confidence limits

Measurement	Mean value I* (± S.D.) II**		Mean % predicted value I* (± S.D.) II**		P value
FVC (l.)	1.23 ± .51	1.32 ± .53	73.4 ±19.1	79.0 ±19.7	< .001
FEV$_{1.0}$ (l.)	0.91 ± .42	1.00 ± .46	63.3 ±15.3	70.0 ±17.9	< .001
MMEF (l./sec.)	0.87 ± .41	1.12 ± .57	48.7 ±17.0	62.0 ±25.1	< .005 > .001
MBC (l./min.)	41.8 ±16.5	44.6 ±16.6	75.9 ±13.9	81.0 ±14.0	< .02 > .01
FEV$_{1.0}$/VC%	69.9 ±11.3	72.0 ±12.0	—		< .3 > .2

*Before bronchodilator administration.
**After bronchodilator administration.

the means and standard deviations are shown in Tables I and II respectively. It can be seen that in the 73 studies there is a small but

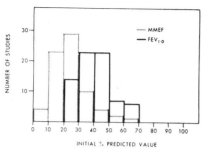

FIG. 4—Initial measurements (73 studies outside the 95% confidence limits for the $FEV_{1.0}$) of the $FEV_{1.0}$ and MMEF expressed as percentages of the predicted normal values.

significant improvement in FVC, MMEF and MBC, an overall increase of 5%. The change in $FEV_{1.0}$ was significant ($P<.02>.01$). Similar small changes occurred with the FVC and MBC measurements in those 22 studies in which the initial airway obstruction was less severe (Table II), but the change in $FEV_{1.0}$ became highly significant ($P<0.001$) and there was a 13% improvement in the MMEF. There is a much larger standard deviation of the post-isoproterenol MMEF value; four studies out of the 22 showed more than a 30% improvement, which accounts for this higher figure.

By giving only the mean changes, we do not show how many patients improved after bronchodilator administration and how many did not. Each individual initial measurement from the group of 73, expressed as a percentage of the predicted normal value, was subtracted from the corresponding result obtained after inhalation of the drug, and the difference or change is plotted in Fig. 5. In the $FEV_{1.0}$ measurements 25 deteriorated and 48 improved. MMEF changes followed a similar pattern but more patients showed a higher percentage of change. Only 14 out of 73 MBC studies showed deterioration rather than improvement.

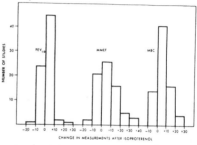

FIG. 5—Change in the percentages of the predicted values before and after bronchodilator administration in the 73 studies in which the initial $FEV_{1.0}$ was outside the 95% confidence limits.

Twenty-seven of the 73 studies included additional tests of functional residual capacity, thoracic gas volume and airway resistance measurements and were analyzed as a sub-group. The individual measurements are recorded in Table III; the means and standard deviations are given in Table IV. There is a large discrepancy between the initial mean FRC as measured by the helium dilution method and by the body plethysmograph, indicating "trapped gas" and hyperinflation. The mean TGV drops by only 90 ml. after isoproterenol. By contrast, the mean airway resistance, expressed as its reciprocal, airway conductance, divided by the thoracic gas volume at which the measurement was made (specific conductance, S_{Gaw})

TABLE III

Lung volume and flow rate measurements in cystic fibrosis

Patient	Age (yrs.)	Height (cm.)	Sex	VC Initial value (l.)	VC I*	VC II**	FEV1.0 Initial value (l.)	FEV1.0 I*	FEV1.0 II**	MMEF Initial value (l./sec.)	MMEF I*	MMEF II**	MBC Initial value (l./min.)	MBC I*	MBC II**	FEV1.0/VC% I#	FEV1.0/VC% II##	FRCHe Initial value (l.)	FRCHe I*	TGV Initial value (l.)	TGV I*	TGV II**	Raw Initial value (cm.H2O/l./sec.)	Raw Change initial value	SGaw Initial value (sec.⁻¹·cm.H2O⁻¹)	SGaw I*	SGaw II**
T.B.	17	163	M	2.55	65	64	1.32	41	34	0.92	23	18	74.8	62	61	52	44	3.25	155	5.01	213	213	4.07	− .46	.049	26	29
,,	17	165	M	2.32	60	68	1.42	43	40	1.04	26	29	63.0	53	53	56	42	4.29	119	4.90	200	193	3.88	− .94	.053	27	37
,,	17	165	M	2.40	62	60	1.07	32	33	0.58	14	12	63.3	53	52	45	43	4.29	183	5.08	216	216	3.74	− .95	.053	27	37
G.L.	10	151	M	2.29	76	69	0.99	37	46	0.83	22	28	65.1	71	82	60	49	1.95	118	2.77	158	147	1.60	+ .69	.226	117	87
,,	10	151	M	1.47	49	50	0.74	28	27	0.71	22	15	69.6	66	83	67	65	1.72	118	2.87	164	172	3.04	− .36	.115	59	64
,,	11	151	M	1.04	35	40	0.78	29	29	0.81	25	29	34.8	36	48	50	56	1.72	104	2.23	135	135	2.65	+ .11	.169	88	84
,,	11	151	M	1.55	52	80	1.07	40	31	0.78	23	24	74.8	75	69	56	69	2.20	133	2.99	171	165	2.35	− .33	.142	74	88
D.B.	12	149	M	2.02	67	65	1.04	40	61	0.79	23	57	82.2	82	99	53	58	2.18	132	2.79	159	159	2.54	− 1.08	.109	73	127
J.R.	8	141	F	1.79	60	79	0.99	43	43	0.73	23	17	67.3	69	63	57	55	1.57	101	1.88	111	107	3.28	− .29	.162	82	94
B.K.	27	165	M	1.84	77	56	1.24	50	52	0.45	17	25	51.5	63	69	55	78	2.08	154	2.05	146	157	5.63	− 2.32	.086	44	71
J.B.	12	149	F	1.70	54	77	0.99	38	43	1.02	25	21	52.9	56	63	55	55	1.24	155	1.66	74	74	6.28	− 2.41	.096	49	79
J.B.	12	154	F	2.06	74	86	1.31	50	46	0.85	26	32	79.4	84	78	60	60	1.86	120	2.04	132	126	6.60	+ .29	.075	38	38
D.B.	10	139	M	2.62	61	68	1.79	64	59	1.12	32	48	76.8	70	70	61	67	2.22	126	2.86	151	145	3.08	+ .13	.114	59	58
D.N.	9	133	M	1.47	58	64	0.99	47	48	0.67	24	30	55.8	79	82	54	45	1.64	114	2.17	161	167	4.78	− 1.05	.096	50	61
C.N.	10	140	F	1.23	33	50	0.56	29	38	0.38	16	23	41.8	67	72	64	71	0.99	90	1.63	138	129	6.61	+ .75	.190	93	84
C.H.	15	143	F	1.16	50	30	0.82	37	35	0.56	20	21	51.5	71	64	66	64	1.29	99	2.01	148	148	9.92	− 1.09	.075	39	48
H. Van D.	15	156	F	0.83	33	60	0.58	25	22	0.31	11	28	42.9	50	52	60	70	1.66	111	2.49	166	166	2.97	− 1.72	.041	21	25
P. McG.	10	138	M	1.76	60	89	1.23	62	70	0.82	25	54	108.6	103	70	72	91	2.89	160	2.92	162	156	9.40	− 3.58	.115	60	74
G.W.	10	133	M	1.95	85	43	1.30	41	67	0.96	36	68	44.5	57	64	60	59	1.41	113	1.41	113	109	7.97	− 2.23	.075	39	64
S. Van D.	12	163	M	0.58	28	65	0.53	28	48	0.55	27	27	35.8	54	91	47	44	1.51	137	2.04	185	191	4.79	− 1.60	.061	31	43
N. McP.	8	125	F	2.58	70	31	1.53	48	28	1.04	27	18	71.3	61	59	65	90	2.20	96	2.63	112	117	12.10	− .92	.079	41	59
M.S.	10	134	M	0.63	43	55	0.43	28	17	0.35	18	15	34.1	53	71	54	76	0.77	79	1.85	191	197	7.06	− .48	.045	23	24
F.T.	24	169	M	0.95	66	72	0.42	52	37	0.25	24	28	46.0	64	73	54	80	1.28	107	1.83	153	148	2.89	− .29	.078	40	44
D.M.	19	168	M	2.84	66	67	1.83	52	58	1.00	24	24	97.0	77	90	62	44	3.01	111	4.07	153	136	4.15	− .60	.060	31	38
D.M.	10	145	M	2.67	62	62	1.45	43	46	0.60	14	15	62.7	73	76	54	56	2.74	101	5.45	202	173	6.13	− 2.76	.044	25	30
V.C.	8	128	F	1.73	67	90	1.11	46	60	0.78	26	50	48.8	55	80	64	62	1.95	134	3.00	205	164	12.63	+ 1.77	.054	28	64
V.C.	8	128	F	0.63	34	35	0.35	21	24	0.22	10	13	23.6	38	44	62	—	1.57	150	2.23	217	189	—	—	.035	18	18

* % predicted value before bronchodilator administration.
** % predicted value after bronchodilator administration.
# FEV1.0/VC% before bronchodilator administration.
FEV1.0/VC% after bronchodilator administration.

TABLE IV
Changes in lung volumes and flow rates after isoproterenol in 19 patients
(27 studies) with cystic fibrosis

Measurement	Mean value I* (± S.D.)	II**	Mean % predicted value I* (± S.D.)	II**	P value
VC (l.)	1.73 ± .68	1.84 ± .70	57.6 ±15.6	61.9 ±16.7	< .005 > .001
FEV$_{1.0}$ (l.)	1.03 ± .40	1.08 ± .42	39.2 ±11.2	41.3 ±13.0	< .2 > .1
MMEF (l./sec.)	0.71 ± .26	0.90 ± .43	23.0 ±10.8	28.6 ±14.4	< .005 > .001
MBC (l./min.)	52.2 ±23.7	66.9 ±21.8	63.9 ±14.1	70.9 ±15.1	< .001
FEV$_{1.0}$/VC%	61.1 ±11.0	59.3 ± 8.2	—	—	< .4 > .3
INITIAL FRC (l.)$_{He}$	2.01 ± .78	—	119.3 ±27.0	—	—
TGV$_p$ (l.)	2.77 ±1.14	2.68 ±1.06	160.1 ±36.3	155.0 ±33.9	< .05 > .025
TGV$_p$-FRC$_{He}$(l.) ("trapped gas")	.76 ± .60	—	—	—	—
S$_{G_{aw}-1}$ (Sec. cm.H$_2$O-1)	.092 ± .049	.114 ± .051	48.2 ±25.4	58.1 ±26.2	< .005 > .001

*Before bronchodilator administration.
**After bronchodilator administration.

increased by 10%, indicating a true alteration in airway conductance. This flow measurement appears to be the most sensitive in demonstrating a change following isoproterenol administration. The individual results of specific conductance before and after broncho-

dilator administration are shown in Fig. 6. When the data for the group are treated as a whole there is no correlation between the initial airway conductance, expressed as airway resistance, and the change produced (r = .231) (Fig. 7); however, when one set of values (patient V.C.) is excluded the correlation becomes significant (r = .579).

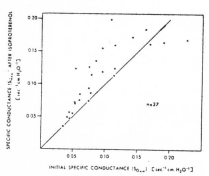

FIG. 6—Relationship of specific conductance before and after bronchodilator administration.

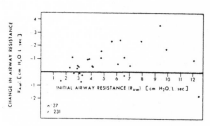

FIG. 7—Initial airway resistance plotted against change in airway resistance, after bronchodilator administration.

Mean initial R$_{aw}$ 5.31 (S.D. ± 2.96)
Mean change R$_{aw}$ -0.74 (S.D. ± 1.11)

Comment

Controversy exists over results of earlier bronchodilator trials on patients with cystic fibrosis. Six patients studied by West, Levin and di Sant 'Agnese[1] had no change in the maximal breathing capacity after Vaponefrin administration. Cook et al.[2] state that in four patients, bronchospasm was not found to be the cause of obstruction since no significant decrease in resistance was demonstrable even when isoproterenol was used in doses large enough to produce tachycardia. In a paper by Beier et al.[3] spirometric values after isoproterenol inhalations were not tabulated since in all 20 patients the drug failed to produce significant changes. Goldring et al.[16] state that Vaponefrin improved the maximal ventilatory capacity in only one patient out of 21 receiving it. This patient also had a history of asthma. Polgar and Barbero[5] showed a mean increase of 5.1% in the $FEV_{1.0}$ and 6.3% in the MBC in six patients, and Royce[17] reported one child whose MBC changed from 29.8 to 51.0 litres per min. (30 to 52% predicted normal) following an unspecified bronchodilator drug.

Lung volume measurements before and after administration of bronchodilator drugs in three separate trials showed small but significant changes; unfortunately, concomitant flow rates were not reported.[14, 18, 19]

We have shown that, statistically, there is an improvement in flow rates of MMEF and MBC in the first group of 73 studies and more especially in the airway conductance in the sub-group of 27,

without any real drop in the functional residual capacity as measured by the body plethysmograph. In 20 instances out of 27 there was an increase in airway conductance (decrease in airway resistance) when the resistance value was corrected for the change in lung volume (Fig. 6).

When the effect of isoproterenol inhalation was measured by a change in R_{aw}, our results suggest that there is a significant correlation between the initial R_{aw} value and the change in R_{aw} after treatment.

All these changes are small, however, compared with those produced by bronchodilator administration to asthmatic children in our laboratory.[20] The most important question remains: has isoproterenol any value in the treatment of cystic fibrosis? Response to the drug varies from patient to patient, and this should determine its use in each individual. The body plethysmograph is an elaborate means for measuring response, and a spirometer is just as satisfactory.

We wish to thank our technicians, Miss A. Liwanag and Mr. N. Tigas, for their help; the Department of Visual Education; Miss S. Hayton for secretarial help; and especially Dr. D. N. Crozier for allowing us to study his patients.

References

1. WEST, J. R., LEVIN, S. M. AND DI SANT 'AGNESE, P. A.: Pediatrics, 13: 155, 1954.
2. COOK, C. D. et al.: Ibid., 24: 181, 1959.
3. BEIER, F. R. et al.: Amer. Rev. Resp. Dis., 94: 430, 1966.
4. MATTHEWS, L. W. et al.: J. Pediat., 65: 558, 1964.
5. POLGAR, G. AND BARBERO, G. J.: Amer. J. Dis. Child., 100: 733, 1960 (abstract).
6. MELLINS, R. B. et al.: Pediatrics, 41: 560, 1968.
7. DUBOIS, A. B. et al.: J. Clin. Invest., 35: 322, 1956.

8. DUBOIS, A. B., BOTELHO, S. Y. AND COMROE, J. H.: *Ibid.*, 35: 327, 1956.
9. KAMEL, M. *et al.*: *Scand. J. Resp. Dis.*, 50: 125, 1969.
10. FEATHERBY, E. A., WENG, T.-R. AND LEVISON, H.: *Arch. Dis. Child.*, 44: 382, 1969.
11. WENG, T.-R. AND LEVISON, H.: *Amer. Rev. Resp. Dis.*, 99: 879, 1969.
12. OPPENHEIMER, E. A., RIGATTO, M. AND FLETCHER, C. M.: *Lancet*, 1: 552, 1968.
13. GOLDBERG, I. AND CHERNIACK, R. M.: *Amer. Rev. Resp. Dis.*, 91: 13, 1965.
14. LIFSCHITZ, M. I. AND DENNING, C. R.: *Ibid.*, 99: 399, 1969.
15. MACKLEM, P. T. AND MEAD, J.: *Arch. Environ. Health (Chicago)*, 14: 5, 1967.
16. GOLDRING, R. M. *et al.*: *J. Pediat.*, 65: 501, 1964.
17. ROYCE, S. W.: Cardiac and pulmonary complications in fibrocystic disease of the pancreas. *In*: Fibrocystic disease of the pancreas, report of the eighteenth Ross Pediatric Research Conference, Ross Laboratories, Columbus, Ohio, 1956, p. 79.
18. MATTHEWS, L. W. *et al.*: *Amer. J. Dis. Child.*, 102: 555, 1961 (abstract).
19. GANDEVIA, B. AND ANDERSON, C.: *Arch. Dis. Child.*, 34: 511, 1959.
20. LEVISON, H., WENG, T.-R. AND FEATHERBY, E. A.: *Annals of the Royal College of Physicians and Surgeons of Canada*, 2: 32, 1969 (abstract).

175

Survival of Patients With Cystic Fibrosis

Nancy N. Huang, MD;
Carlos N. Macri, MD;
Joseph Girone, MD;
and Ann Sproul, MD

Fifteen years ago the measures current in management of patients with cystic fibrosis consisted simply of intermittent antibiotic therapy and addition of pancreatic enzymes and vitamins to the diet. In 1957, at St. Christopher's Hospital for Children, a cystic fibrosis clinic was established to provide close follow-up study and long-term antibiotic therapy, and the use of aerosol

medication was introduced. Since 1962, with support from the Commonwealth of Pennsylvania, from the state of New Jersey, and from the National Cystic Fibrosis Research Foundation, a program of intensive care has evolved which embraces intensive antibiotic therapy, aerosol therapy, mist tent care, physical therapy, early administration of measles vaccine, and improved dietary management in young infants. These changes have markedly improved the general comfort and outlook of these patients. In order to determine whether such intensive care

Read before the ninth annual Cystic Fibrosis Club meeting, Atlanta City, NJ, April 30, 1968.

has enhanced the long-term survival of these patients, we carried out the study here reported.

Material and Methods

The survival rates of patients admitted to this hospital in three, five-year periods extending from July 1952 to June 1967 were computed according to the "life table method," as described by Cutler and Ederer.[1] The method is one that allows the use of all survival information accumulated up to the closing date of a period. In computing the five-year survival rate and its standard error the method is not restricted to patients who were observed over the entire period, but it also utilizes valuable information contributed by patients who came under observation four, three, two, and even one year prior to the closing date. The three groups of our patients comprise:

1. Group 1 consisted of 37 patients admitted between July 1952 and June 1957, inclusively. We chose December 1957 as the closing date for the analysis of their survival rate.

2. Group 2 consisted of 73 patients admitted between July 1957 and June 1962, for whom we chose December 1962 as the closing date for the analysis of survival rate.

3. Group 3 consisted of 129 patients admitted between July 1962 and June 1967, for whom December 1967 was chosen as the closing date.

Those patients who survived the first 5½-year period were not included in the analysis of patients admitted in the subsequent periods; nor were group 2 survivors entered in the analysis of group 3 patients. Similarly, patients admitted in the period between July 1952 and June 1957 who died after December 1957 were not included in the analysis of the survival rate of patients in the subsequent periods, nor were group 2 deaths occurring after December 1962 charged to group 3. Accordingly, there are three separate cohorts in this study. Patients with meconium ileus are included; three each in group 1 and group 2 and five in group 3.

Results

Age and Sex Distribution.—Table 1 shows the sex of the patients studied and the age on entry into the study. Sixty percent of patients coming under observation in the first study period were under 1 year of age, and 38% and 39% of the patients in periods 2 and 3 were under 1 year of age. The age distribution of patients first seen in period 2 is comparable to that of patients in period 3. There were more male than female patients in period 1, equal incidence of the two sexes in period 2, and significantly more female than male patients in period 3. More female infants and preschool girls first entered observation in period 3.

Comparison of Survival Rates (Table 2 Through 4 and Fig 1).—Patients in group 1 had significantly lower survival rates during intervals of one to five years after first observation than patients in group 2 and 3. The survival rates at intervals of 1 to 4 years after admission were significantly better also for group 3 patients than for group 2 patients. The five-year survival rate of patients in group 2 and 3 were not significantly different from each other, but the trend favors group 3 patients. In group 1, the high mortality in the first two years of observation is evident. In group 2 and group 3 patients there was definite improvement in survival rates, with marked reduction of mortality of group 3 patients in the first four years of observation, after which the mortality began to creep up. The five-year survival for group 3 patients is better than for group 2

Table 1.—Age and Sex Distributions on First Observation of the Patients in Three Study Periods

Age Range (Yr)	Period 1 (1952 to 1957)				Period 2 (1957 to 1962)				Period 3 (1962 to 1967)			
	M	F	No.	%	M	F	No.	%	M	F	No.	%
0–1	15	7	22	60	15	13	28	38	16	34	50	39
>1–3	3	2	5	14	9	9	18	25	8	17	25	19
>3–5	1	3	4	11	5	6	11	15	7	10	17	13
>5–10	5	1	6	16	5	8	13	18	13	14	27	21
>10	0	0	0	0	3	0	3	4	4	6	10	8
Total	24	13	37	101	37	36	73	100	48	81	129	100

Table 2.—Pertinent Data and Survival Rates of Three Groups of Patients With Cystic Fibrosis

	Period 1 July 1952 to June 1957	Period 2 July 1957 to June 1962	Period 3 July 1962 to June 1967
Total No. of patients	37	73	129
Total deaths	21	22	16
Cumulative survival rates from first observation through intervals of:			
1 yr	54.5% ± 8.1%	82.9% ± 4.5%	95.2% ± 1.9%
2 yr	35.0% ± 8.7%	76.4% ± 5.1%	92.4% ± 2.4%
3 yr	35.0% ± 8.7%	63.6% ± 6.4%	89.8% ± 2.9%
4 yr	35.0% ± 8.7%	63.6% ± 6.4%	85.6% ± 4.0%
5 yr	35.0% ± 8.7%	63.6% ± 6.4%	76.6% ± 7.0%

patients, but the difference is not statistically significant.

Survival Rates According to Sex Distribution of Group 2 and 3 Patients (Table 5).—The five-year survival rate for female patients was higher than that for male patients in group 2, but no significant sex difference was found in the survival rates of group 3 patients.

Survival Rates According to the Severity of Pulmonary Involvement on First Observation in Group 2 and 3 Patients (Table 6).—The severity of pulmonary involvement of these

patients was arbitrarily divided into the following two categories in order to maintain a sufficient number of patients in each category for comparison.

Mild and Moderate.—This group consists of patients whose developmental status placed them between the third and 95th percentiles in respect to weight and height, who sustained normal activity for age, had infrequent or no cough, inconstant moist rales on physical examination, and early or no clubbing of fingers, and whose pulmonary

178

Table 3.—Illustration of Computation of the Five-Year Survival Rate and Its Standard Error of Group 3 Patients

(1) Years of Follow-Up Study to X + 1	(2) Alive at Beginning of Interval l_x	(3) Died During Interval d_x	(4) Lost to Follow-Up During Interval u_x	(5) Withdrawn Alive During Interval w_x	(6) Effective Number Exposed to the Risk of Dying (Column 2 − ½ Column 4 − ½ Column 5) l'_x	(7) Proportion Dying (Column 3 ÷ Column 6) q_x	(8) Proportion Surviving (1 − Column 7) p_x	(9) Cumulative Proportion Surviving From Diagnosis Through End of Interval ($p1 \times p2 \ldots \times px$) P_x	(10) (Column 6 − Column 3) $l'_x - d_x$	(11)* (Column 7 ÷ Column 10) $q_x / l'_x - d_x$	SE
0–1	129	6	0	6	126	0.048†	0.952	0.952	120	0.0004	1.9%
1–2	117	3	0	32	101	0.030	0.970	0.924	98	0.0003	2.4%
2–3	82	2	0	23	70.5	0.028	0.972	0.898	68.5	0.0004	2.9%
3–4	57	2	1	27	43	0.047	0.953	0.856	41	0.0011	4.0%
4–5	27	2	0	16	19	0.105	0.895	0.766	17	0.0062	7.0%
5–6	9	1	0	8	...	...	...	...	...	...	...

* Square root of sum of number in column 11 multiplied by the 5-year survival rate yields the SE for the five-year survival rate. Other standard errors are computed in the same way.

† The figures are rounded off to three digits below decimal for the Table.

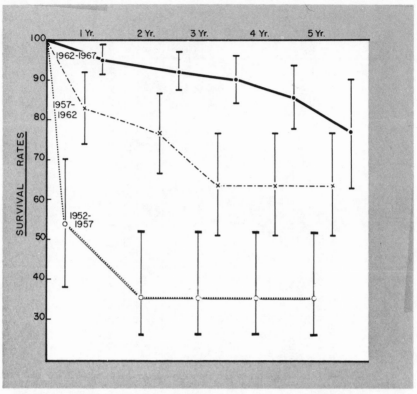

Fig 1.—Cumulative survival rates and 95% confidence limits (**vertical lines**) of patients with cystic fibrosis followed from first observation through intervals of 1 to 5 years during period of 1952 to 1957 (**open circles** and **dotted line**). 1957 to 1962 (**crosses** and **broken line**), and 1962 to 1967 (**closed circles** and **solid line**).

findings ranged from nearly normal to moderate overaeration, with or without transient confluent densities on the roentgenograms of the chest.

Advanced.—This group of patients presented weight and height below the third percentile, poor exercise tolerance, constant cough, constant rales and abnormal breath sounds, clubbing of fingers, and persistent confluent densities, localized or generalized, on radiologic examination.

There were proportionately more mild or moderately ill patients in group 3. The survival rates of such patients were approximately the same in groups 2 and 3. The marked increase in four-year survival for group 3 patients with advanced pulmonary disease over group 2 patients is significant but five-year survival rates in group 2 and 3 patients with advanced disease are not significantly different.

Survival Rates of Group 2 and Group 3 Patients According to Age on First Observation (Table 7).—Patients whose disease was diagnosed after 1 year

Table 4.—Comparison of Survival Rates of Groups 1 and 2 and 2 and 3, Respectively

Years of Survival	Group 1 and 2 Observed Difference ± SE of Difference	p	Group 2 and 3 Observed Difference ± SE of Difference	p
1	28.4% ± 9.5%	<0.01	12.3% ± 5%	<0.01
2	41.4% ± 10%	<0.001	16.0% ± 6%	<0.01
3	28.6% ± 10%	<0.01	26.2% ± 7%	<0,001
4	28.6% ± 10%	<0.01	22.6% ± 7%	<0.001
5	28.6% ± 10%	<0.01	13.0% ± 9.5%	>0.1 (Not significant)

Table 5.—Cumulative Survival Rates of Group 2 and 3 Patients According to Sex Distribution

	Group 2		Group 3	
	M	F	M	F
Total No. of patients	37	36	48	81
Total deaths	14	8	6	10
Cumulative survival rates from first observation through intervals of:				
1 yr	74.0% ± 8.1%*	91.6% ± 4.5%*	98.0% ± 2.1%*	93.6% ± 2.8%*
2 yr	74.0% ± 8.1%	82.2% ± 6.4%	93.2% ± 3.8%	92.0% ± 3.1%
3 yr	54.0% ± 9.8%	74.0% ± 7.7%	87.1% ± 5.4%	89.7% ± 3.9%
4 yr	44.0% ± 10.9%	74.0% ± 7.7%	82.4% ± 6.7%	85.8% ± 5.3%
5 yr	44.0% ± 10.9%	74.0% ± 7.7%	82.4% ± 6.7%	69.5% ± 11.2%

* Survival rates ± SE.

Table 6.——Cumulative Survival Rates of Group 2 and 3 Patients According to Severity of Pulmonary Involvement on First Observation

	Group 2		Group 3	
	Mild-Moderate	Advanced	Mild-Moderate	Advanced
Total No. of patients	41	32	90	39
Total deaths	3	19	4	12
Cumulative survival rates from first observation through intervals of:				
1 yr	100%	61.8% ± 7.2%*	98.9% ± 1.1%*	86.6% ± 5.4%*
2 yr	96.9% ± 3.0%*	51.8% ± 8.9%	97.5% ± 1.7%	80.6% ± 6.6%
3 yr	88.4% ± 6.2%	35.0% ± 8.8%	95.5% ± 2.5%	71.7% ± 8.3%
4 yr	88.4% ± 6.2%	35.0% ± 8.8%	92.6% ± 3.9%	63.2% ± 10.7%
5 yr	88.4% ± 6.2%	35.0% ± 8.8%	92.6% ± 3.9%	21.2% ± 17.5%

* Survival rates ± SE.

Table 7.——Cumulative Survival Rates of Group 2 and 3 Patients According to Age on First Observation

	Group 2		Group 3	
	Age < 1 Yr on First Observation	Age > 1 Yr on First Observation	Age < 1 Yr on First Observation	Age > 1 Yr on First Observation
Total No. of patients	28	45	47	82
Total deaths	10	12	8	8
Cumulative survival rates from first observation through intervals of:				
1 yr	76.5% ± 8.2%*	86.1% ± 5.3%*	89.3% ± 4.5%*	97.5% ± 0.2%*
2 yr	67.6% ± 9.0%	80.7% ± 6.2%	84.8% ± 5.6%†	97.5% ± 0.2%†
3 yr	61.5% ± 10.1%	67.5% ± 8.0%	84.8% ± 5.6%	90.9% ± 3.9%
4 yr	61.5% ± 10.1%	67.5% ± 8.0%	79.8% ± 7.3%	87.2% ± 5.1%
5 yr	61.5% ± 10.1%	67.5% ± 8.0%	79.8% ± 7.3%	73.8% ± 9.5%

* Survival rates ± SE.
† The difference between these two survival rates is significant statistically, $P < 0.05$. All the other differences in survival rates are not significant on statistical analysis.

of age had higher survival rates in both group 2 and 3 than those whose disease was diagnosed before 1 year of age. In each age range, the survival rate of group 3 patients was higher than that of group 2 patients, but the differences were not statistically significant, except for two-year cumulative survival rates of group 3 patients.

Table 8.—Cumulative Survival Rates of Group 3 Infants First Observed at Birth or at 2 to 6 Months of Age

	Group 3 Infants First Observed at Birth	Group 3 Infants First Observed at 2 to 6 Mo of Age
Total No. of Patients	19	16
Total deaths	2	5
Cumulative survival rates from first observation through intervals of:		
1 yr	94.6% ± 5.3%	81.3% ± 9.8%
2 yr	88.1% ± 9.0%	74.5% ± 11.0%
3 yr	88.1% ± 9.0%	74.5% ± 11.0%
4 yr	88.1% ± 9.0%	62.5% ± 14.6%
5 yr	88.1% ± 9.0%	62.5% ± 14.6%

Survival Rates of Group 3 Infants Diagnosed at or Shortly After Birth vs Those Diagnosed at 2 to 6 Months of Age (Table 8).—Infants whose condition was diagnosed at or shortly after birth, before the onset of respiratory symptoms, showed better survival than those first seen between 2 and 6 months of age, after the onset of respiratory symptoms, but the small number of patients does not permit any confident inference.

Survival of Patients With Meconium Ileus.—All three infants in group 1 and two of three infants in group 2 died within four weeks after neonatal surgery. The remaining infant of group 2 and all five infants of group 3 survived postoperatively and continue to do well in the 5-year follow-up study.

 Comment

We have shown how the life table method of Cutler and Ederer[1] lends itself to the analysis of the survival rate of patients with cystic fibrosis. The method is simple and permits comparison of treatment programs adopted in successive periods of time.

We found a definite and progressive improvement in survival rate over the past 15 years. Our results follow the same trend as those of others.[2-4] Warwick and Monson[2] constructed their life tables according to the age of the patients on first observation and computed the life expectancies of their cohorts. This method is much different from ours, and it is not possible to make a comparison.

Young and Jackson[3] computed annual case fatality during the period of 1958 to 1965 but disregarded the duration of follow-up study. Therefore, it is not possible to compare their rates with our results calculated by the life table method. Anderson[4] did not give a detailed description of her method, but it seems to be similar to the method adopted for this study. Her five-year cumulative survival rate to June 1965 of 111 patients admitted during the period of 1958 to 1962 was about 60%, a figure approximately the same as we obtained in our group 2 patients. Our group 3 patients observed from July 1962 through December 1967 had a better survival rate than Anderson's

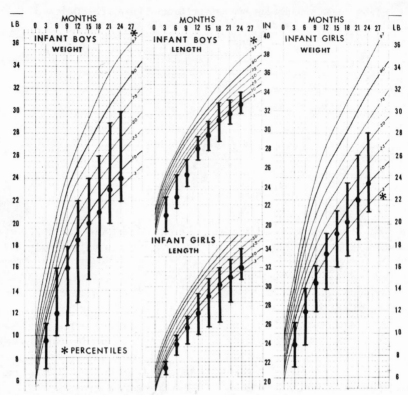

Fig 2.—Range, median height and weight of infants seen in 1957 to 1962 as plotted on Stuart percentile grid. (From Sproul and Huang[5])

patients observed to June 1965.

The patients in our group 1 were mostly young infants with advanced pulmonary involvement. Many did not survive the initial period of hospitalization. Those who did survive did not have the advantage of a supervised home care program. In 1957, our cystic fibrosis program was organized, and most of the patients were under the direct supervision of one of us (N.N.H.). Since then, we feel that a program of systematic care and regular evaluation, with more intensive use of antibiotic therapy,

has led to distinct improvement in the survival rate. Since 1962, further changes have occurred:

1. The extension to patients with cystic fibrosis of the Crippled Children's Program of the Commonwealth of Pennsylvania and of the State of New Jersey has greatly relieved their families of the major burden of drug cost and clinic fees. This has made it easier for the patients to be followed closely for therapeutic evaluation.

2. Mist tent and aerosol therapy have been made available to the ma-

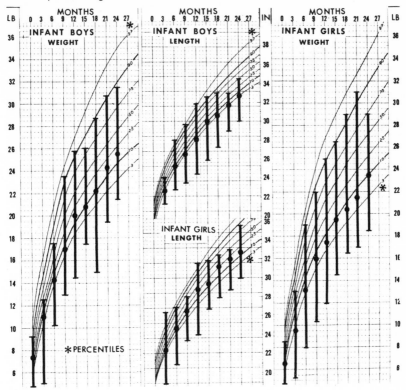

Fig 3.—Range, median height and weight of infants seen in 1962 to 1967 as plotted on Stuart percentile grid.

jority of patients through the local chapters of the National Cystic Fibrosis Research Foundation.

3. New antibiotic agents have become available, principally the semisynthetic penicillins and cephalosporins. These are effective against staphylococci and certain gram-negative organisms and can be used for prolonged periods of time with relatively low toxicity. They have been used parenterally during periods of clinical exacerbation of disease. For long-term maintenance therapy of patients with advanced and moderate disease, we also use semi-

synthetic penicillins by oral administration with or without the addition of chloramphenicol or tetracyclines.

4. The importance of physical therapy and postural drainage has been emphasized to parents.

5. Live attenuated measles vaccine has been universally employed.

6. More cases have been diagnosed before the onset of serious respiratory involvement.

7. A well organized program of home care has been established for most of the patients under the supervision of public health nurses.

The above factors have contributed

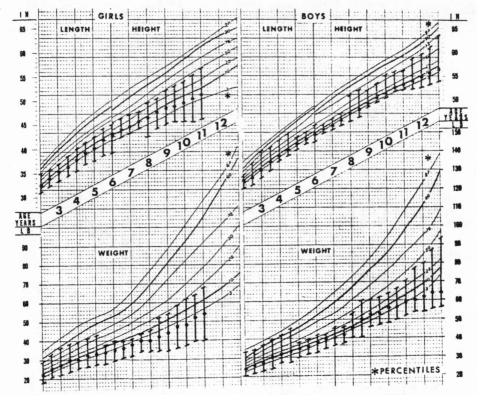

Fig 4.—Range, median height and weight of children (2 to 13 years) seen in 1957 to 1962 as plotted on Stuart percentile grid. (From Sproul and Huang[5])

greatly toward the improved survival rate of our group 3 patients. It is difficult to tell which factor is most important. Certainly, the severity of pulmonary involvement on first observation, the age when diagnosis is made and the therapy instituted, and an aggressive approach in combatting bacterial infections by the proper use of antibiotic agents plus energetic bronchial drainage are of utmost importance in prolonging the lives of these patients.

Our colleagues in this field often attribute the improved outlook of patients with cystic fibrosis to physical therapy and bronchial drainage and disregard the effect of antibiotics. We are certainly impressed by the effectiveness of the antibiotics especially in the management of patients with advanced disease and during acute exacerbations. Physical therapy and bronchial drainage contribute greatly to the success of treatment but must be used concurrently with antibiotic therapy in patients with evidence of active infection. Most of our moderately-ill patients and all of our severely-ill

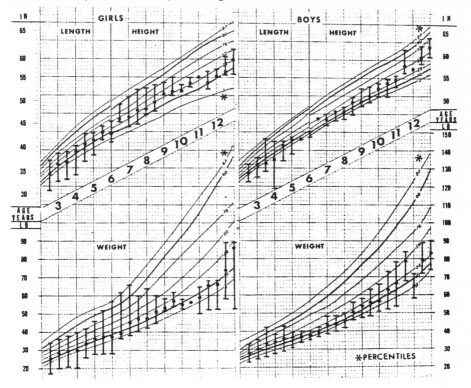

Fig 5.—Range, median height and weight of children (2 to 13 years) seen in 1962 to 1967 as plotted on Stuart percentile grid.

patients are on continuous antibiotic administration, physical therapy, postural drainage, aerosol inhalation, and mist tent at night. Patients with a mild disease certainly do not require continuous administration of antibiotics, and some patients receive none at all. We often have a problem with patients of older age whose condition has been newly diagnosed. They cannot sleep in a mist tent at night, nor will they ac-

cept physical therapy. Some of them will only take antibiotics. These patients generally do well on antibiotics alone, and we are satisfied with their progress.

Our group 3 patients not only survived longer but also lived a relatively better life than group 2 patients. Our previous study showed positive correlation between severity of pulmonary disease and growth retardation in patients with cystic fibrosis.[5]

Therefore, a comparison of growth rate of group 2 patients with that of group 3 patients should provide enough evidence of the effectiveness of our intensive care program for group 3 patients. We published the growth pattern of 50 children who were followed in the period of 1957 to 1962 (group 2).[5] Recently, we analyzed the growth records of 105 patients followed in 1962 to 1967 (group 3). Comparison of the growth patterns as illustrated in Fig 2 through 5 shows improvement in ranges and median weights and heights of female infants of group 3 over female infants of group 2 and significant improvement in weights of male infants of group 3 over male infants of group 2. Older patients (2½ to 13 years) of group 3 have median weights and heights at or above the tenth percentile of normals from male and female patients, whereas the median weights and heights of group 2 patients are below the tenth percentile. The weight curve for group 3 male patients did not exhibit a plateau at about 10 years of age as was observed in group 2 patients. However, the growth curve of female patients is noted to reach a plateau at approximately age 10 years. It has been the general belief that female adolescents with cystic fibrosis have a more severe disease than the male adolescents. This certainly is true with respect to growth patterns, but the present study shows no distinct sex difference in survival rates.

The fact that patients whose condition was diagnosed after 1 year of age had better survival rates than those whose condition was diagnosed under 1 year of age suggests that those who survive early infancy without specific treatment have a milder disease than others. Those patients whose disease is diagnosed under 1 year of age after the onset of respiratory symptoms are generally very sick, and the mortality is high. Therefore, establishment of the diagnosis and of a plan of management within the first year of life is crucial; to do so within the first 6 months may be even more critical. Only two of 19 infants in this study died where diagnosis was made shortly after birth, before onset of respiratory symptoms; the deaths of these two infants were due to fulminating acute gastroenteritis. On the other hand, five of 16 patients died who were observed after onset of respiratory symptoms, at 2 to 6 months of age; all died of respiratory insufficiency. Since it is important to establish the diagnosis as early as possible, all infants with meconium ileus and all those born in families in which cystic fibrosis has occurred must be tested immediately after birth. If there is any doubt after repeated sweat tests, the infant should be treated as having cystic fibrosis until proven otherwise.

Additional support for early institution of treatment comes from comparison of the growth curves of 19 infants treated before the onset of respiratory involvement with those of 16 infants diagnosed after the onset of respiratory involvement. The median weights of the former group were between the tenth and 75th percentiles, whereas, in the latter group, these weights were all below the tenth percentile.

For all infants where diagnosis was made shortly after birth before the onset of respiratory symptoms, we generally recommend a full prophylactic regimen including pancreatic enzyme supplementation, vitamin administration, mist tent, and physical therapy in addition to antibiotics. This type of prophylactic approach does not prevent the infants from developing respiratory symptoms but can prevent the occurrence of severe pneumonia, pulmonary insufficiency, cor pulmonale, and hypoproteinemia, which being the most serious complications of the disease are associated with a high mortality. It seems to be important to give vitamins and pancreatic enzyme supplementation as soon after birth as possible, but the role of mist tent, physical therapy, and antibiotics before the onset of respiratory symptoms is not yet clear.

As more potent but less toxic antimicrobial agents are discovered, as more effective nebulizing equipment becomes available, and as more trained professionals exhibit interest in the disease, there is reason to anticipate an increasingly encouraging outlook for the patients.

Figure 2 and 4 are reproduced with permission from the *Journal of Pediatrics* (**65**:664-676, 1964).

This investigation was supported in part by Public Health Service research grant FR75, and Center grant from the National Cystic Fibrosis Research Foundation.

Arthur Itkin, MS, and Shirley Braverman, MS, helped with the statistical evaluation, Kung-tse Sheng, MD, and Varuni Promadhat, MD, gave clinical assistance, and Samuel L. Cresson, MD, George P. Pilling, III, MD, and Lawrence A. Somers, MD, referred their patients with meconium ileus to our cystic fibrosis follow-up study.

The artwork was done by Chung Yu Liu and Yun Yong.

References

1. Cutler SJ, Ederer F: Maximum utilization of the life table method in analyzing survival. *Chronic Dis* **8**:699-712, 1958.

2. Warwick WJ, Monson S: Life table studies of mortality, *Modern Problems in Pediatrics*. Berne, Switzerland, S Karger, in Rossi E, Stoll E (eds): vol 10, pp 353-367, 1967.

3. Young WF, Jackson ADM: The prognosis of cystic fibrosis, in Rossi E, Stoll E (eds): *Modern Problems in Pediatrics*. Berne, Switzerland, S Karger, vol 10, pp 350-352, 1967.

4. Anderson CM: Long term study of patients with cystic fibrosis, in Rossi E, Stoll E (eds): *Modern Problems in Pediatrics*. Berne, Switzerland, S Karger, vol 10, pp 344-349, 1967.

5. Sproul A, Huang N: Growth patterns in children with cystic fibrosis. *J Pediat* **65**:664-667, 1964.

MARTIN I. LIFSCHITZ
CAROLYN R. DENNING

QUANTITATIVE INTERACTION OF WATER AND CYSTIC FIBROSIS SPUTUM[1]

The use of continuous nebulization for the treatment of bronchopulmonary disease, popularized by Denton[2,3] and others in the early 1950s, entered a new era with the introduction in the mid-1960's[4] of high density mist produced by ultrasonic nebulizers. Such units were capable of emitting large volumes of relatively uniform and stable water droplets with a mean diameter of less than 10 μ. It was assumed that evaporation would further reduce particle size, permitting delivery of generous amounts of water to the smaller airways. Indeed, there were many reports of success with ultrasonic mist in terms of sputum liquification and restoration of airway patency.[4,5] One of the most impressive areas of application appeared to be mist tent therapy of patients with cystic fibrosis.[6]

Reports of the clinical efficacy of mist tent therapy are at variance with recently published theoretic considerations of the quantity of water deposited in the lower respiratory tract by such therapy. Matthews and co-workers[6-8] reported significant benefit in patients with cystic fibrosis from the use of mist tents, especially with ultrasonic mist. This benefit was manifest both by immediate improvement in pulmonary function,[6,7]

and by increased survival over a prolonged period.[8] Avery and associates,[9] and Wolfsdorf and co-workers[10] challenged the rationale of mist therapy, calculating that the maximum amount of water that could be deposited below the larynx during a 24-hour period of ultrasonic mist therapy would be only 49 ml in an adult. Matthews and Doershuk,[11] in turn, challenged the experimental design of the study on which these calculations were based. Baker and Griffiths[12] pointed out the many difficulties and pitfalls of speculative reasoning in this area.

One facet of the problem that appears to have escaped consideration is the question of how much water is required per unit volume of sputum to effect a significant reduction in viscosity?

The assumption has been made that deposition in the lower respiratory tract of 49 ml of water per 24 hours, or 16 ml during eight hours in a mist tent, is insignificant.[10] Yet there are no quantitative data available on the interaction of water and sputum on which to base realistic estimates of the effects of varying volumes of water. The present study was designed to provide such data for the purulent, highly viscous sputum of patients with cystic fibrosis.

Sputum was collected from patients with cystic fibrosis by expectoration into a plastic cup. Patients had not received aerosol or mist treatment for at least three hours before collection. Specimens were collected over a 20- to 60-minute period and frozen until studied. According to Lie-

1 Supported by a grant from the National Cystic Fibrosis Research Foundation.

2 Denton, R., and Smith, R. M.: Amer. J. Dis. Child., 1951, 82, 433.

3 Denton, R.: Dis. Chest, 1955, 28, 123.

4 Andrews, A. H.: Proceedings of the First Conference on Clinical Applications of the Ultrasonic Nebulizer, DeVilbiss Co., Somerset, Pennsylvania, 1966.

5 Abramson, H. A.: Proceedings of the Second Conference on Clinical Applications of the Ultrasonic Nebulizer, DeVilbiss Co., Somerset, Pennsylvania, 1967.

6 Doershuk, C. F., Matthews, L. W., Gillespie, C. T., Lough, M.D., and Spector, S.: Pediatrics, 1968, 41, 723.

7 Matthews, L. W., Doershuk, C. F., and Spector, S.: Pediatrics, 1967, 39, 176.

8 Doershuk, C. F., Matthews, L. W., Tucker, A. S., Nudelman, H., Eddy, G., Wise, M., and Spector, S.: J. Pediat., 1964, 65, 677.

9 Avery, M. E., Gulina, M., and Nachma, M. D.: Pediatrics, 1967, 39, 160.

10 Wolfsdorf, J., Swift, D. L., and Avery, M. E.: Pediatrics, 1969, 43, 799.

11 Matthews, L. W., and Doersuk, C. F.: Pediatrics, 1969, 43, 902.

12 Baker, H., and Griffiths, J. C.: Amer. Rev. Resp. Dis., 1968, 97, 1136.

berman,[13] a single freezing and thawing has no effect on sputum viscosity.

Viscosity was measured with an eight-speed rotational viscometer[14] incorporating a cone and plate spindle arrangement and a circulating constant temperature bath at 37° C. The method used was that described by Lieberman,[13] except that the cone plate gap was set at 0.0025 inch and readings were recorded manually.

Specimens were measured at 1, 2.5, or 5 rpm; the speed was selected to give the highest reading without going off scale. Some extremely viscid specimens gave readings that were off scale even at 1 rpm and could not be used for study.

To establish a base line, the sputum sample was rotated at a constant speed for five minutes, and readings were taken every minute. A few specimens apparently had a very high elastic component and would not remain in the cup, but rolled up into a gumlike mass and crept above the cone. Such specimens had to be discarded because a valid baseline could not be obtained.

After a base line viscosity was established distilled water equal to 10, 20, 30, or 40 per cent of the volume of sputum in the cup was added to the specimen, and the mixture was rotated again at the same constant speed. Viscosity readings were taken every minute during a ten-minute period, and the specimen was discarded. Ten separate specimens were studied at each of the four dilutions.

Variation of relative viscosity with time of the sputum is shown in figure 1. The control curve represents the mean values of ten sputum samples rotated for 15 minutes without the addition of water. Viscosity readings were stable after five minutes of spin and did not decrease during the subsequent ten-minute period.

Each of the lower four curves represents the mean values of a series of ten different sputum analyses. The decrease in sputum viscosity after addition of water was complete within one minute and viscosity remained stable thereafter.

In figure 2 are shown the mean relative viscosities one minute after the addition of the various volumes of water to the sputum. The response to the addition of water was essentially linear over the range studied.

* * *

Distilled water has a viscosity-reducing effect on sputum from patients with cystic fibrosis that is rapid, complete in one minute, and directly

[13] Lieberman, J.: Amer. Rev. Resp. Dis., 1968, 97, 654.

[14] Wells Brookfield Micro Viscometer, Model RVT, Brookfield Engineering Laboratories, Stoughton, Massachusetts.

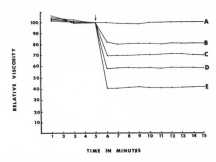

Fig. 1. Viscosity as a function of time in a rotational viscometer for a control sputum specimen (A) and sputum specimens from patients with cystic fibrosis. After 5 minutes, water was added in a volume equal to 10 per cent (B), 20 per cent (C), 30 per cent (D), and 40 per cent (E) of the volume of sputum in the viscometer cup. Each curve represents the mean of ten different sputum analyses.

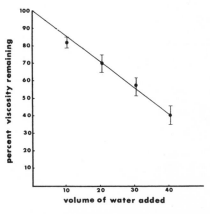

Fig. 2. Mean relative viscosities of sputum specimens after addition of a volume of water equal to 10 per cent, 20 per cent, 30 per cent, or 40 per cent of the sputum volume. The vertical lines extending from each point represent ± SD.

proportional to the volume of water added, characteristics compatible with a simple dilutional mechanism. The magnitude of the effect is such that 1 ml of water can reduce the viscosity of 3 ml of sputum by approximately 50 per cent.

An adult-size patient sleeping eight hours in an ultrasonic mist tent could, according to Wolfsdorf's calculations, deposit 16 ml of water in his lower respiratory tract, or enough to halve the viscosity of 50 ml, almost two ounces, of sputum. The amount of sputum produced daily by patients with cystic fibrosis varies from patient to patient. Some patients do not expectorate at all; others cough up only three or four plugs a day, whereas those with advanced bronchiectasis can produce two or more ounces of sputum daily. How much sputum is swallowed, and how much of the expectorated volume is saliva, are unknown. In a smaller patient, the volume of water deposited would be less, but the volume of sputum to be liquified would also be proportionately less.

From the present data, it can be anticipated that many patients with cystic fibrosis would benefit from ultrasonic mist therapy, even if the volumes of water deposited in the lower respiratory tract were as small as Wolfsdorf has calculated.

In summary: *In vitro* measurements of the effect of water on the viscosity of sputum from patients with cystic fibrosis revealed that the decrease in viscosity was directly proportional to the volume of water added. One ml of water reduced the viscosity of 3 ml of sputum by approximately 50 per cent, suggesting that even small amounts of water deposited in the lower respiratory tract could have significant clinical effect.

Complications

Neonatal Jaundice Associated With Cystic Fibrosis

William F. Taylor, MD, and
Boulos Y. Qaqundah, MD

While both focal and generalized cirrhosis of the liver are
common autopsy findings in older
children with cystic fibrosis, early
jaundice and abnormal liver function
are uncommon. We are reporting an
infant with cystic fibrosis whose predominant signs were jaundice and
failure to thrive at 3½ weeks of age.

Report of a Case

On March 25, 1969, a 6-week-old girl was
referred to Orange County Medical Center
by a Public Health Nurse because of failure to thrive and jaundice. Jaundice was
first noticed when the child was 3½ weeks
old. The patient's admission weight was
2,750 gm (6 lb 1 oz) while her birth weight
was 2,865 gm (6 lb 5 oz). The mother reported no cough, abnormal stools, or rectal
prolapse. The mother's first pregnancy terminated eight weeks prematurely with a
still birth. Her second pregnancy produced
a girl who is now 2 years old, living and
well. The patient was the result of a full
term pregnancy, born by uncomplicated la-
bor and delivery. Apgar score was 9 at one
minute. No jaundice or other abnormal
signs were noted in the nursery and the infant and mother were discharged on the
third day after delivery. The infant was
given a commerical formula (Similac) and
by the time of admission, the mother had
added cereal and fruit. Neither chronic
pulmonary disease nor gastrointestinal
disease was present in the family history.

Physical examination revealed a thin infant who appeared chronically ill. There was little subcutaneous fat; edema was not noted. She was alert, had a lusty cry and a voracious appetite. Her skin was warm and dry with a greenish-yellow hue and the sclerae were jaundiced. The liver, palpable 4 cm below the right costal margin, was smooth, nontender, and the edge was easily outlined. The spleen extended 2 cm below the left costal margin. Auscultation of the chest failed to reveal cardiac or pulmonary abnormalities. Stools were firm and clay colored.

Laboratory tests disclosed the following values: mother's blood, O positive; baby's blood, A positive; direct Coombs' test, negative; hemoglobin, 13.1 gm/100 ml; hematocrit, 36%; white blood cell count, 20,800/cu mm; polymorphonuclear leukocytes, 37%; lymphocytes, 51%; monocytes, 10%; eosinophils, 2%; reticulocytes, 2.5%; red blood cell morphological features, normal; bilirubin: total, 6 mg/100 ml, direct, 5 mg/100 ml; VDRL test for syphilis, negative; enzymes: serum glutamic oxaloacetic transaminase, 170 units; serum glutamic pyruvic transaminase, 50 units; alkaline phosphotase, 8.8 Bodansky units; prothrombin time, 80%; stool: pH, 6; bile pigments, negative; urine: white blood cell count, 20 to 30/cu mm; culture of urine by suprapubic tap, no growth; cytomegalic inclusion bodies, negative. Roentgenograms of the chest and skull were normal; intravenous pyelogram was normal.

At this point, a diagnosis of congenital atresia of the bile ducts neonatal hepatitis was thought to be most likely. Subsequently, the possibility of cystic fibrosis was considered. Three sweat chloride determinations by iontophoresis all yielded results greater than 100 mEq/liter. Mist tent therapy and pancreatic enzyme replacement were instituted. Stools gradually returned to a soft consistency and normal color. One week after admission, no jaundice remained, birth weight was regained and three weeks later the patient was discharged. On discharge her weight was 3,260 gm (7 lb 3 oz) and the previously abnormal levels of liver enzymes and bilirubin were normal, while the liver re-

mained palpable 3 cm below the right costal margin. At home, the infant continued to sleep in a mist tent and receive pancreatic enzymes. At 11 months of age, she weighed 6,038 gm (13 lb 5 oz) and her height was 67.3 cm (14 in); both measurements are near the third percentile. The liver was 2 cm below the right costal margin; the spleen was not palpable and levels of liver enzymes and serum bilirubin mained normal. The mother reported no symptoms of gastrointestinal or respiratory disease.

Comment

In children with cystic fibrosis, liver fibrosis has been found histologically[1] at 1 week of age, which suggests the possibility of intrauterine involvement.[2] Yet, elevated levels of liver enzymes and hepatic symptoms seldom occur until late in the disease. di Sant' Agnese and Blanc[3] emphasized that liver function and bilirubin level remain normal because cirrhosis is focal and adequate hepatic parenchyma remains until late in the disease process.

Our patient and two other neonates[2,4] with cystic fibrosis have been described with jaundice and abnormal results of liver function studies. In 1965, Gatzimos and Jowitt[4] reported four cases of cystic fibrosis presenting as jaundice in infancy. At autopsy, they found bile plugs in the biliary system of all their patients. Porta et al[1] surgically biopsied the liver, pancreas, and gall bladder in five infants with cystic fibrosis who were neither jaundiced nor suffering from clinical liver disease. The most common finding was cholangiolar proliferation thought to be secondary to mucus inspissation.

Although our patient was not submitted to liver biopsy, it seems logical from the course to assume that bile or mucus plugs caused the jaundice, abnormal enzyme levels, and hepato-megaly. It also seems logical that by some unknown mechanism this obstruction was relieved and resulted in complete resolution of the clinical and laboratory signs of liver disease. The reversibility of this child's clinical symptoms suggests that a choleretic such as tocamphyl may be efficacious in treating the neonate with jaundice secondary to cystic fibrosis.

It is impossible to prove that our patient did not suffer from neonatal hepatitis since a specific test is unavailable. The limited period of jaundice and the diagnosis of cystic fibrosis, which is known to affect the liver in neonates, make the diagnosis of neonatal hepatitis unlikely. This infant has fared better than the two previously reported neonates with cystic fibrosis and jaundice. One of them had jaundice at 4 days of age and died at the age of 2 weeks, while the other had jaundice at 10 days of age, esophageal varices at 1 year, and died at 3 years of age.

This investigation was supported in part by Regional Medical Programs, Area VIII grant 1-G03-RM-00019-01.

Nonproprietary and Trade Names of Drug

Tocamphyl—*Gallogen, Syncuma.*

References

1. Porta EA, Stein AA, Patterson P: Ultra structural changes of the pancreas and liver in cystic fibrosis. *Amer J Clin Path* 42:451-465, 1964.
2. Shier KJ, Horn RC: The pathology of liver cirrhosis in patients with cystic fibrosis of the pancreas. *Canad Med Assoc J* 89:645-651, 1963.
3. di Sant' Agnese PA, Blanc WA: A distinctive type of biliary cirrhosis of the liver associated with cystic fibrosis of the pancreas. *Pediatrics* 18:387-409, 1956.
4. Gatzimos CD, Jowitt RH: Jaundice in musociscidosis (fibrocystic disease of pancreas). *Amer J Dis Child* 89:182-186, 1955.

Complications of iodide therapy in patients with cystic fibrosis

Thomas F. Dolan, Jr., M.D., and Lewis E. Gibson, M.D.

O N E   O F   many medications used for therapy of patients with cystic fibrosis of the pancreas is iodide in some form. To date there are no reports concerning the efficacy of iodides or their side effects in such patients. The complications of iodide therapy observed at the Yale–New Haven Hospital Cystic Fibrosis Clinic are described.

METHODS

Charts of 110 patients with cystic fibrosis

Supported in part by grants from the National Cystic Fibrosis Research Foundation and from the Health Department of the State of Connecticut.

Presented in part at the Eleventh Annual Cystic Fibrosis Club meeting at the Marlborough-Blenheim Hotel, Atlantic City, April 29, 1970.

were reviewed. All patients were diagnosed by determination of sweat electrolytes and the presence of typical clinical findings. Fifty-five patients had received daily iodide therapy for at least one year, usually much longer, and 55 patients had not been given iodides. The age range of the patients receiving iodides was 18 months to 21 years. All of the patients were examined by the authors during the years 1966 through 1969. An effort was made to determine the time of onset of goiter, if present, and the presence of signs and symptoms of hypothyroidism, rhinorrhea, or nasal polyps. Fifty patients received iodide as a sodium salt in a dose of 15 to 30 mg. of iodine per kilogram of body weight, and 5 patients received 1 to 2 mg. of iodide per kilogram of body weight as an organic iodide.

T3 uptake by red cells was performed on sera of 38 patients on one or more occasions by a modification of the conventional method.[1] In addition, a small sampling of T3 uptake by red cells was performed on sera of patients not receiving iodide. In our laboratory butanol extractable iodine levels were found to be elevated in sera from patients receiving high doses of iodide and were not a reliable index of thyroid function.[1]

RESULTS

No goiters were noted in the 55 patients with cystic fibrosis not receiving iodides, and all T3 uptakes were within normal limits in those patients so studied. Goiters occurred in 46 of 50 children receiving sodium iodide and in 1 of 5 patients receiving organic iodide. The earliest occurrence of a goiter was 3 months after onset of treatment; the usual time was 2 to 3 years. In one patient a goiter did not appear until 12 years after institution of iodide therapy. In all cases the thyroid was visibly enlarged, diffusely symmetric, nonnodular, and occasionally tender. Eighteen of the thyroid glands were at least 4 times normal size and were cosmetically disfiguring; 17 glands were estimated to be 3 times normal size, and 11 were twice normal size.

Hypothyroidism. Nine of 34 children receiving sodium iodide had abnormal T3 uptake values in the hypothyroid range; all had goiters. The duration of iodide therapy preceding the T3 uptake test was 2 to 9 years, with an average of 4½ years. Four of the 9 with abnormal T3 uptake had clinical evidence of hypothyroidism; an additional 3 children receiving sodium iodide had clinical signs of hypothyroidism with goiters but no tests of thyroid function were performed. Two of 5 children receiving organic iodide had abnormal T3 uptakes, one of whom had clinical hypothyroidism; neither of these 2 patients had a goiter.

Among the 8 children with clinical hypothyroidism, the following signs or symptoms were present: cold intolerance, 8 of 8; coarse and thickened skin, 5 of 8; coarse and thickened hair, 5 of 8; massive alopecia, 3 of 8; and puffy face, 4 of 8. In all instances treatment with thyroid extract resulted in prompt improvement of signs and symptoms of hypothyroidism within 8 weeks. The thyroid gland returned to normal size within 6 months in all patients with goiters except 2 whose glands remained enlarged for 3 years before finally returning to normal size.

Rhinorrhea and polyps. Rhinorrhea was defined as severe when it was copious in degree and almost constant; rhinitis was considered severe when the patient or his parents complained of an almost continuously stuffy nose without nasal discharge. Thirty-four of 55 patients receiving iodide therapy had rhinorrhea or rhinitis but in all instances this preceded iodide therapy and was not apparently worsened by iodides. Rhinorrhea or rhinitis occurred in 11 of 40 patients not receiving iodide (15 of these 55 patients were lost to follow-up). Fourteen children receiving iodide developed nasal polyps, usually 4 or 5 years after institution of iodide therapy. The age of appearance of the first polyp was 4 to 10½ years; no polyps were observed in any child receiving iodides for less than 4 years. To date no children not receiving iodides have developed polyps, even with rhinorrhea or rhinitis; only 3 of these patients are over 3 years of age, however. There was a strong history of allergy in either the patient or his parents in 11 of the 14 children who developed nasal polyps, as compared with an over-all incidence of personal or family history of allergy of only 18 per cent of the entire Cystic Fibrosis Clinic population.

Other side effects. No excess lacrimation or acne was noted; 2 children had to discontinue iodide therapy because of generalized skin rashes; two discontinued treatment because of gastrointestinal disturbances. Several other patients complained of mild gastrointestinal upset but discontinuation of medication was unnecessary.

DISCUSSION

In 1961, Oppenheimer and McPherson[2] reported a case of iodide-induced goiter and reviewed 23 previously reported cases. In 1963, Begg and Hall[3] described 23 iodide-induced goiters and collected 65 more from the literature. A possible mechanism whereby iodides in large doses may produce hypothyroidism was described by Wolff and Chaikoff.[4] In animal studies iodide in excess doses was trapped by the thyroid but failed to combine with tyrosine, leading to a failure of T3 and T4 synthesis. Braverman and Ingbar[5] have shown that prolonged administration of iodide results in an adaptive decreased thyroidal uptake preventing accumulation of excess iodide in the thyroid and allowing production of hormone. Presumably hypothyroidism and goiter occur when this homeostatic mechanism does not function.[6, 7]

The occurrence of goiter in 85 per cent of patients with cystic fibrosis receiving iodides suggests either that many of these patients have an unusual sensitivity to the goitrogenic effects of iodide or that iodide, if given long enough and in sufficient doses, will produce goiter and hypothyroidism in any patient. Begg and Hall[3] suggest that the latter is true. Falliers and associates[8] reported an incidence of 4 per cent moderate to marked goiter and 14 per cent minimal thyroid enlargement, all within 3 to 6 weeks of initiation of therapy in asthmatic children. There are no reports of long-term iodide therapy with reference to goiter formation in patients with cystic fibrosis.

The occurrence of polyps only in patients who had previously received iodides is curious. This may be due to the age distribution of the patients studied, as most of the children with rhinorrhea not receiving iodides are under 3 years of age. It had been the policy of the clinic to begin iodide therapy in all children when a diagnosis of cystic fibrosis was made. Only 2 of 50 patients with cystic fibrosis and nasal polyps reported by Schwachman and associates[9] were under 4 years of age at the time of the first observed polyp. It would appear that in patients with a history of allergy and pre-existing chronic rhinorrhea or rhinitis, the administration of iodide may enhance the development of nasal polyps since rhinorrhea is a well-known side effect of iodide therapy.

Efficacy of iodides. No attempts were made to study the effects of iodides in reference to the sputum volume or viscosity in this population; such studies are extremely difficult to perform. Although iodides have been used for many years, there are very few data to document their efficacy. Goodman and Gilman[10] state that they act by stimulating bronchial secretions. Several authors claim improvement in some asthmatic children.[8, 11] Animal studies[12] have shown that iodide is secreted into the bronchi but studies[13-16] purporting to show volume or viscosity changes in sputum give conflicting results; most claims as to their usefulness are based on clinical impressions. Recently Lieberman and Kurnick[17] have suggested that iodides help to liquify purulent sputum by enzymatic induction of proteolysis from polymorphonuclear cells. Possibly this is beneficial but there are no studies showing improvement in pulmonary function tests of patients with chronic pulmonary disease receiving iodides. Since concluding this study we have discontinued the use of iodides in our clinic and are planning studies to evaluate their efficacy.

Many of the signs of iodide toxicity or iodide-induced hypothyroidism such as rhinorrhea, submaxillary gland swelling, delayed pubescence, fatigue, lethargy, depression, constipation, and failure to grow properly are similar to those seen in children with cystic fibrosis. The absence of a goiter does not exclude the presence of hypothyroidism; 2 patients receiving organic iodides developed this complication without a goiter.

REFERENCES

1. Seligson, D., and Hillman, E.: Clinical laboratories, Yale–New Haven Hospital. Personal communication.
2. Oppenheimer, H. J., and McPherson, H. T.: The syndrome of iodide induced goiter and myxedema, Amer. J. Med. 30: 281, 1961.
3. Begg, T. B., and Hall, R.: Iodide goiter and

hypothyroidism, Quart J. Med. **32:** 351, 1963.

4. Wolff, J., and Chaikoff, I. L.: Plasma in organic iodide as homeostatic regulator of thyroid function, J. Biol. Chem. **174:** 555, 1948.

5. Braverman, L. E., and Ingbar, S. H.: Changes in thyroidal function during adaptation to large doses of iodide, J. Clin. Invest. **42:** 1216, 1963.

6. Braverman, L. E., and Woeber K. A.: Induction of myxedema by iodide in patients euthyroid after radioiodine or surgical treatment of diffuse toxic goiter, New Eng. J. Med. **281:** 816, 1969.

7. Harrison, M. T., Alexander, W. D., and Harden, R. McG.: Thyroid function and iodine metabolism in iodine-induced hypothyroidism, Lancet **1:** 1238, 1963.

8. Falliers, C. J., McCann, W. P., Chai, H., Ellis, E. F., and Yazdi, N.: Controlled study of iodotherapy for childhood asthma, J. Allerg. **38:** 183, 1966.

9. Shwachman, H., Kulczycki, L. L., Mueller, H. L., and Flake, C. G.: Nasal polyposis in patients with cystic fibrosis, Pediatrics **30:** 389, 1962.

10. Goodman, L. S., and Gilman, A. Z.: The pharmacologic basis of therapeutics, ed. 3, New York, 1965, The MacMillan Company, pp. 811-815.

11. Siegal, S.: The asthma suppressive action of potassium iodide, J. Allerg. **35:** 252, 1964.

12. Gordonoff, T.: Les expectorants et l'expectoration, Ann. med. **38:** 249, 1935.

13. Palmer, K. N.: Sputum liquifiers, Brit. J. Dis. Chest **60:** 177, 1966.

14. Hillis, B. R., and Stein, L.: The assessment of expectorant drugs, Scottish Med. J. **3:** 252, 1958.

15. Forbes, J., and Wise, F.: Expectorants and sputum viscosity, Lancet **273:** 767, 1957.

16. Schiller, L. W.: Bronchial asthma—views on therapy, New Eng. J. Med. **269:** 94, 201, 1963.

17. Lieberman, J., and Kurnick, N. B.: The induction of proteolysis in purulent sputum by iodides, J. Clin. Invest. **43:** 1892, 1964.

200

AUTHOR INDEX

KEY-WORD TITLE INDEX

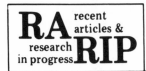

RA recent articles &
research **RIP** in progress

Guide to Current Research

The research summaries appearing in the following section were obtained through a search of the Smithsonian Science Information Exchange data base conducted in July, 1973.

The Exchange annually registers 85,000 to 100,000 notices of current research projects covering a wide range of disciplines and sources of support. SSIE endeavors to retain up to two full years of current research information in its active file. The selection of summaries appearing in this section does not represent the complete SSIE collection of information on this topic, but, rather, has been specifically tailored to reflect the scientific content of this particular volume. A limited number of summaries may have been omitted because clearance for publication by the supporting agency or organization was not received prior to the publication date.

SSIE is the only, single source for information on ongoing and recently terminated research in all areas of the life, physical, behavioral, social and engineering sciences. The SSIE file is updated daily by a professional staff of scientists utilizing a comprehensive and flexible system of hierarchical indexing. Retrieval of subject information is conducted by these same specialists, using computer-connected, video display terminals which allow instant access to the entire data base and on-line refinement of search strategies. SSIE offers an information service unequalled anywhere: comprehensive and vital information on who is conducting what research where and under whose support.

More current information, and in some cases expanded coverage, on the topic considered in this volume is available directly from SSIE. This information is offered at modest cost in the form of custom searches of the SSIE file designed specifically to meet the user's need or as an update of the subject search in this section. For more information on SSIE, contact MSS or write directly to the Smithsonian Science Information Exchange, 1730 M Street, N.W., Washington, D.C. 20036. Subject search or updated package requirements may be discussed with SSIE scientists by calling the Exchange at (202) 381-5511.

CHEMISTRY OF MUCIN IN CYSTIC FIBROSIS,
O.P. BAHL, State University of New York,
School of Medicine, Buffalo, New York 14214

This work has as its objective the characterization of highly purified mucins isolated from the submaxillary secretions of normal children and patients with cystic fibrosis. A major motivation is the determination of whether the mucins secreted by exocrine glands are or are not "abnormal" in the patient with cystic fibrosis. The work will be initiated with mucins isolated from the submaxillary secretions because of the ready availability of these secretions, and the indication in the literature that they are altered in patients with the disease. Special emphasis will be placed on physical chemical studies of the mucins, and on the structure of the carbohydrate moieties of the mucin. Should results warrant, the investigations will be extended to the symptom-free families of patients. Parallel studies will be carried out with submaxillary secretions from the dog in an effort to define the regulatory processes governing synthesis and secretion of submaxillary mucin.

CYSTIC FIBROSIS IDENTITY OF THE PLASMA
FACTOR,
S.H. BISHOP, Baylor University, School of
Medicine, Houston, Texas 77025

The average life expectancy for the patient with cystic fibrosis is 21 years. The disease is hereditary and homozygous recessive. Symptoms develop from birth. One common feature in the etiology of the disease is the presence of a factor in the plasma, sweat, and saliva which interferes

with salt balance in normal tissues. This
plasma factor has not been isolated and
characterized. Nothing is known concerning
the origin of the disease or the plasma
factor. Present methods of screening for
the early detection of the disorder and for
heterozygous conditions are not quantitative
(accurate). The purpose of this study is
four-fold: (a) the isolation in pure form
of some of this plasma factor, (b) the
preparation of an antibody to the plasma
factor and development of an immune assay
for the plasma factor, (c) preparation of a
large quantitiy of the plasma factor using
the quantitative immune assay, and (d)
preliminary chemical characterization of the
factor. If the correlation between presence
of the factor in the plasma and the disease
state is absolute, then the antibody will be
used as the basis for a quantitative immune
assay for rapid and accurate detection of
the disease state.

MUCIN SECRETION BY RESPIRATORY EPITHELIAL
EXPLANTS,
T.F. BOAT, Case Western Reserve Univ.,
School of Medicine, Cleveland, Ohio 44106

It is the objective of this study to
compare mucins secreted by respiratory
epithelium of children who have chronic
obstructive pulmonary disease (COPD), e.g.,
cystic fibrosis, bronchial asthma, and
asthmatic bronchitis, with mucins secreted
by age and sex-matched control subjects.
Respiratory tract secretions are usually
either inaccessible or grossly contaminated;
we have therefore developed an organ culture
system for long-term maintenance of human
respiratory epithelium and collection of its
uncontaminated secretory product. Mucins,
electrophoretically and chromatographically

similar to those secreted in vivo, can be
harvested from culture medium in amounts
sufficient to permit fractionation and
detailed chemical analysis. Experiments are
proposed to refine the culture methodology
and thereby insure maximal and consistent
mucin secretion. These experiments will be
evaluated by histochemical and
radioautographic studies, and by
quantitation of macromolecules secreted
daily into the medium. When optimal culture
conditions have been established, explant
mucins will be collected, dialyzed,
solubilized by reduction and
carboxymethylation, and fractionated by
standard chromatographic and electrofocusing
techniques, or on immuno-absorbent columns
containing insolubilized lectins.
Carbohydrate and sulfate content, amino acid
composition, oligosaccharide structure and
linkage to the polypeptide chain, blood
group activity, and virus hemagglutinin
inhibition activity will be determined for
each purified mucin. Chemical analyses of
purified mucin(s) secreted in vitro and in
vivo will be compared to insure that major
alteration of explant mucin has not
occurred. If similarity is demonstrated,
the composition of purified mucin(s)
secreted by explants from normal subjects
and subjects with COPD will then be
compared. We anticipate that molecular
differences will be identified and
ultimately related to the underlying
pathogenetic mechanism in one or more of
these diseases.

HOST RESPONSE IN CYSTIC FIBROSIS TO
PSEUDOMONAS SLIME,
J.R. BORING, Emory University, School of
Medicine, Atlanta, Georgia 30322

Pulmonary infection caused by

Pseudomonas aeruginosa growing in the tracheobronchial tree of children with cystic fibrosis is one of the most serious problems in the clinical management of these patients. Methods for prevention of infection or eradication of the organism are seldom successful.

Infections which are especially persistent are established by mucoid strains of Ps. aeruginosa, organisms which produce copious amounts of slime on artificial media. Studies in our laboratory have indicated that Pseudomonas slime is antiphagocytic when added to mixtures of rabbit leukocytes and Ps. aeruginosa. The effect of slime is abolished when multivalent antiserum (against cells and slime) is added to mixtures. These observations suggest that the persistence of mucoid strains may reflect an immunological tolerance to the slime polysaccharide in children with cystic fibrosis.

The objective of this project is to understand the host-pathogen relationship between mucoid Ps. aeruginosa and patients with cystic fibrosis. To accomplish this we wish to determine: 1) The numbers of mucoid organisms usually present in the sputum; 2) the extent of slime formation in vivo by mucoid strains; and 3) whether patients form antibodies (circulatory or secretory) against the slime of the strain they harbor.

The degree of colonization will be estimated by enumeration of organisms both in direct smears of sputum and by plate count of viable bacteria. Whether slime is formed in vivo will be confirmed by examination of sputum using the indirect-fluorescent-antibody technique with hyperimmune antiserum prepared against slime. Whether circulatory antibodies (IgG or IgM) are produced by children against slime will be examined using the complement fixation test. The presence of secretory

antibody in the sputum will be determined
using the indirect fluorescent antibody
test.

CHARACTERIZATION OF THE CYSTIC FIBROSIS
SERUM FACTOR,
B.H. BOWMAN, Univ. of Texas, School of
Medicine, Galveston, Texas 77550

The oyster cilia assay detects
homozygous and heterozygous cystic fibrosis
(CF) genotypes. The serums of CF
homozygotes and heterozygotes contain a
factor which causes ciliary cessation in
oyster gills. The inhibitor has now been
partially purified from serums of CF
heterozygotes and homozygotes. Biochemical
characterization has revealed that the CF
ciliary inhibitor is, or is bound to, a
gamma G immunoglobulin molecule with a
molecular weight of approximately 200,000.
The inhibitory fraction has been isolated by
ion exchange chromatography, rivanol
precipitation, gel filtration, immunosorbent
columns and preparative starch block
electrophoresis. Results from papain
digestion and immunofluorescence indicate
that the CF factor is not an autoantibody.
Electron microscopy data demonstrate an
atypical coiling of cilia after exposure to
CF serum. This request is for support to
complete the characterization of the ciliary
inhibitor and to determine its malfunction
in CF patients. The site of action of the
ciliary inhibitor present in the bod fluids
of CF individuals will be sought by
immunofluorescence and ferritin labelled
antibody techniques. The ciliary inhibitor
produced in CF lymphocyte grown in culture
containing radioactive amino acids will be
characterized structurally. This protein
will be contrasted to its normal counterpart

synthesized in cell lines from non-CF individuals. It seems likely that the ciliary inhibitor is, or is close to, the primary defect of the CF gene since asymptomatic heterozygotes demonstrate ciliary inhibition in their serums when tested by the oyster cilia assay. Designating the properties, malfunction and site of action of the basic defect of CF will permit the development of specific therapy for patients with cystic fibrosis.

STUDY OF AN EXTRINSIC NON-RENAL RENIN-ANGIOTENSIN SYSTEM IN MAN, R.A. CAMPBELL, Univ. of Oregon, School of Medicine, Portland, Oregon 97201

This study will acquire information concerning the status of what we shall call the "extrinsic" renin-angiotensin system of the pulmonary, gastrointestinal, and exocrine gland systems of normal children and those with hypertension, nephrotic syndrome and cystic fibrosis. Inasmuch as the renin-angiotensin system "extrinsic" to the renal apparatus/adrenal glomerulosa axis may play a significant role in the ontogenetic and philogenetic development of extra-renal ion transport control, the status of such a proposed extrinsic renin-angiotensin system merits careful evaluation. There are cogent and compelling experimental and clinical reasons for undertaking a detailed analysis of both the renal and the extrinsic renin-angiotensin systems in the above- named pathological states.
        Using radioimmunoassay techniques with high sensitivity, renin levels of activity, angiotensin I and angiotensin II concentrations will be determined in the blood, urine and exocrine secretions of

normal and diseased children. In addition, converting enzyme activity and angiotensinase activity will be determined on selected biological samples.

GASTROINTESTINAL STUDIES IN CYSTIC FIBROSIS, P.A. DISANTAGNESE, U.S. Dept. of Hlth. Ed. & Wel., P.H.S. Natl. Insts. of Health, Bethesda, Maryland 20014

It is well known that patients with cystic fibrosis may develop hepatic biliary cirrhosis which may lead to significant clinical problems during life. Serologic tests for liver function in children have been difficult to interpret because of the lack of good normal data in this age group. Alkaline phosphatase in particular is known to increase markedly during adolescence secondary to active bone growth, thus making interpretation of this test as a measure of liver function most difficult. We have examined the sera from normal children and cystic fibrosis patients in an attempt to: 1) establish new norms for serologic liver tests in children; 2) demonstrate the age-independency of the liver isoenzyme of alkaline phosphatase; 3) establish the incidence of serologic evidence of liver disease in cystic fibrosis.

It has been reported that orally administered L-arginine is beneficial in decreasing the amount of steatorrhea, abdominal pain, and improving weight gain in patients with cystic fibrosis. It also has been suggested that oral administration of bicarbonate (NaHCO3) may improve the malabsorption associated with pancreatic insufficiency due to other causes. In view of these findings, a study was undertaken to investigate the efficacy of orally administered L-arginine and NaHCO3 in the

210

treatment of malabsorption due to cystic fibrosis.

Little has been written about about the x-ray abnormalities of the duodenum and small bowel in cystic fibrosis. Abdominal pain of obscure etiology is a relatively common sympton in cystic fibrosis, and a high incidence of duodenal ulcers has been reported for patients. Barium studies of the duodenum and upper gastrointestinal tract were undertaken to further study these clinical manifestations.

TISSUE CULTURE STUDIES IN CYSTIC FIBROSIS, P.A. DISANTAGNESE, U.S. Dept. of Hlth. Ed. & Wel., P.H.S. Natl. Insts. of Health, Bethesda, Maryland 20014

In view of our previous reports concerning increased glycogen stores by cystic fibrosis fibroblasts, an attempt was made to investigate glucose uptake and utilization by fibroblasts from cystic fibrosis patients and normals. Questions to be answered with fibroblast experiments include: 1) what are the comparative uptake and diffusion of glucose by the cell; 2) what are the effects of insulin and fetal calf serum on glucose transport; 3) what changes of stored glycogen occur during the life cycle of the cell; 4) are there morphologic differences between cystic fibrosis and normal cells; 5) is the "CF factor" present either within the cell or in the growth-supporting media; 6) can other biochemical abnormalities (e.g. methylation of RNA) be demonstrated in the CF cell?

CLINICAL STUDIES IN CYSTIC FIBROSIS,
P.A. DISANTAGNESE, U.S. Dept. of Hlth. Ed. &
Wel., P.H.S. Natl. Insts. of Health,
Bethesda, Maryland 20014

The prevailing opinion has been that
males with cystic fibrosis are sterile due
to aspermia secondary to abnormal
mesonephric derivatives. The existence of
fertile males with this disease would have
obvious genetic, social, psychological, and
therapeutic implications. The semen from
two fertile male patients was studied
chemically and morphologically.

The improved life expectancy of
patients with cystic fibrosis has been
associated with an increased frequency of
certain complications, some of which have
considerable prognostic significance.
Pulmonary parameters rather than nutritional
and dietary aspects currently appear to be
associated with prognosis. A need has
arisen for a systematized scoring system
based as much as possible on objective
criteria; such a system could be used to
prognosticate and as a uniform and
consistent method of evaluating and
following patients for clinical purposes and
studies. Previous scoring systems have been
more subjective and have not considered
these newer complications. A new scoring
system and mortality curve were devised.

As more patients with cystic fibrosis
are reaching adulthood, it has become
important to assess psychological as well as
physical performance and to determine how
these patients can best be helped to
function well. Therefore, an in-depth
psychiatric evaluation was made of
adolescents and young adults with cystic
fibrosis.

FLOW RATES & ELECTROLYTES IN MINOR SALIVARY
GLAND SALIVA IN NORMAL SUBJECTS & PATIENTS
WITH CYSTIC FIBROSIS (ABBREV),
P.A. DISANTAGNESE, U.S. Dept. of Hlth. Ed. &
Wel., P.H.S. Natl. Insts. of Health,
Bethesda, Maryland 20014

A new method for extracting saliva from
small salivary glands from the inner aspect
of the upper lip was devised. This method
allows for the first time determination of
sodium, potassium, calcium, and magnesium,
as well as flow rates.
It is notable that minor salivary
glands are the only exocrine gland system in
addition to the eccrine sweat glands that
consistently manifest the sodium abnormality
in cystic fibrosis. In addition, as shown
by the normal values for calcium in the
patients tested in this study, the sodium
defect appears to be independent of the
increased concentration of calcium, as
recently postulated for sweat glands by
other authors.

BIOCHEMICAL STUDIES IN CYSTIC FIBROSIS,
P.A. DISANTAGNESE, U.S. Dept. of Hlth. Ed. &
Wel., P.H.S. Natl. Insts. of Health,
Bethesda, Maryland 20014

The basic defect in cystic fibrosis
remains unknown. Recently several
investigators have described the presence of
two factors in saliva, sweat, and serum of
patients: a ciliary inhibitory factor and a
factor which inhibits sodium reabsorption
across various membranes. Since there is no
easy, reproducible assay for either factor,
studies were done to develop a biologic
assay for the sodium inhibitory factor.
Knowing the time of appearance and

213

origin of amniotic fluid amylase may allow
for the detection of pancreatic deficiency
in utero in cystic fibrosis. This may be of
significance for the antenatal diagnosis of
this disease. Additionally, knowing the
prenatal course of cystic fibrosis may allow
one to apply certain therapeutic procedures
(in the future) antenatally in correcting
basic lesions of this disease.

Several recent reports by other
investigators have implied that the basic
abnormality in cystic fibrosis may be
related to the immunologic system,
particularly IgA. Studies were done to
determine if IgA production by intestinal
mucosa was related to pancreatic deficiency.
If it is, then it may not be related to the
primary etiologic cause of cystic fibrosis.
Therefore, patients with cystic fibrosis and
hereditary pancreatitis (both with
pancreatic insufficiency) were studied.

METABOLIC STUDIES IN CYSTIC FIBROSIS,
P.A. DISANTAGNESE, U.S. Dept. of Hlth. Ed. &
Wel., P.H.S. Natl. Insts. of Health,
Bethesda, Maryland 20014

Comprehensive metabolic studies have
been undertaken with the object of
clarifying the physiopathology of cystic
fibrosis and thus permitting a more
effective and rational approach to prognosis
and treatment. Under study have been
aldosterone metabolism in cystic fibrosis,
calcium metabolism in this disease, and
malabsorption studies in this disorder.

STUDY OF CYSTIC FIBROSIS OF THE PANCREAS,
Z. DISCHE, Columbia University, School of
Medicine, New York, New York 10032

There will be an investigation of
possible changes in the structure of
glycoproteins in the stromata of red cells
of cystic fibrosis patients as a possible
clue to the defect in the pumping mechanism
of cellular surfaces in these diseases. An
investigation will be also conducted on the
possible influence of the presence of
sulfated glycoproteins in mucous secretion
and their influence on physical properties
of these secretions. An influence of
possible A vitamin deficiency on the
physical properties and chemical structures
of glycoproteins of mucous secretions will
be also studied.

SWEAT GLAND DEFECT IN PANCREATIC FIBROSIS,
R.A. ELLIS, Brown University, Graduate
School, Providence, Rhode Island 02912

Eccrine sweat glands in surgical skin
biopsies from normal children and patients
afflicted with pancreatic cystic fibrosis
are studied and compared. Cytochemical, and
electron microscopic techniques are used to
study the localization of specific enzymes
and the sites of synthesis and fate of
glycoproteins and mucopolysaccharides.
Routine electron microscopy of each case
available provides information on cell types
affected by the disease and alterations in
duct and secretory segments of the sweat
glands. Consistent findings in accumulated
data are correlated with other biochemical
and physiological observations.
Studies on other model systems
involving cation secretion are effected on

215

the nasal glands of reptiles and birds.

STUDY OF NBT DYE TEST IN SELECTED CHILDHOOD
DISORDERS,
R.D. FEIGIN, Washington University, School
of Medicine, Saint Louis, Missouri 63110

The nitroblue tetrazolium (NBT) dye
test has been shown to be a valuable aid in
the differential diagnosis of febrile
disorders in immunologically competent,
healthy children and adults. The usefulness
of the test in neonates, children with
malignancy, individuals with sickle cell
disease, or cystic fibrosis, and in steroid
recipients has not been evaluated in detail
and the few studies performed to date have
been relatively limited in scope and yielded
conflicting results. It is particularly
important to determine the validity of the
NBT dye test in these individuals for it has
been well established that they are
compromised with respect to the manner in
which they cope with infection, making
rapidity and accuracy in the diagnosis of
infection essential. We intend to study the
NBT dye test in each of these patient groups
under well controlled conditions. In the
event that the NBT dye reducing ability of
the white blood cells is compromised in the
face of active infection in any of these
disorders, additional insight into the
mechanism for NBT dye reduction will be
sought by performing oxygen consumption
studies and evaluating hexose
monophosphatase shunt activity utilizing a
radioisotopic procedure. These studies
should provide information concerning the
pathogenesis of infection within these
compromised hosts.

SERUM ANTIHYALURONIDASE TITRES IN CYSTIC
FIBROSIS OF THE PANCREAS,
G.E. GIBBS, Univ. of Nebraska, School of
Medicine, Omaha, Nebraska 68105

Purpose: To determine whether in
cystic fibrosis of the pancreas there is an
increased serum antihyaluronidase titre, in
response to increased hyaluronidase, in
response to increased hyaluronic acid
compound.
    Subjects: Children, adolescents, with
and without cystic fibrosis, irrespective of
sex.
    Methods: Determination of serum
antihyaluronidase titres. Determination of
significance of mean difference between
serum antihyaluronidase titres in the two
groups.
    Findings: Lower serum
antihyaluronidase values in cystic fibrosis
than in controls.

SCREENING OF NEWBORNS BY MECONIUM ALBUMIN
FOR CYSTIC FIBROSIS,
G.E. GIBBS, Univ. of Nebraska, School of
Medicine, Omaha, Nebraska 68105

Purpose: To determine practicality of
screening technique with 1 to 30 dilution of
meconium and use of Albustix.
    Subjects: 4,000 newborn infants.
    Methods: All newborns in six hospitals
being tested. Newborns showing more than 30
mg. per 100 c.c.'s albumin to be further
investigated.
    Findings: No CF turned up in 400
infants.

217

METABOLISM OF LYMPHOCYTES IN CYSTIC FIBROSIS,
G.E. GIBBS, Univ. of Nebraska, School of
Medicine, Omaha, Nebraska 68105

Purpose: Verification and exploration
of biochemical abnormality in cultured
lymphocytes in cystic fibrosis.
Subjects: Adolescents, male and
female, with or without cystic fibrosis, 20
patients.
Methods: Lymphocytes are cultured with
determination of total beta-glucuronidase
and chromatographic fractions of it; also
effects of ATPase on conversion of one
fraction to another.
Findings: Beta-glucuronidase in
cultured lymphocytes separate into two
fractions by DEAE chromatography and salt
gradient.   The pregradient form converts to
the gradient form by action of ATPase; the
beta glucuronidase from CF cells converts
more readily than from normal cells.

MODE OF PANCREATIC ENZYME REPLACEMENT,
G.E. GIBBS, Univ. of Nebraska, School of
Medicine, Omaha, Nebraska 68105

Purpose: To determine optimal timing
and effect of accompanying alkali in
effectiveness of pancreatic enzyme therapy.
Subjects: 50 Children and adolescents
aged 2 to 20 years, male and female with
cystic fibrosis.
Methods: Patients in outpatient visits
instructed to take pancreatin before meals
or after meals also before meals with
alkali. Also investigation of individual
meals with I 131 trioleum.

Observation of effect on weight gain.
Similar observations for effect of
bicarbonate or other antacid in alternate
periods along with pancreatin before meals.

Findings: No definite effect from
timing of pancreatin or administration of
alkali. Use of radioactive trioleum with
counting of residual radioactivity in stools
appears to be a satisfactory technique.

BETA-GLUCURONIDASE AND RNA OF
PHYTOHEMAGGLUTININ-STIMULATED CULTURED
LYMPHOCYTES IN CYSTIC FIBROSIS,
G.E. GIBBS, Univ. of Nebraska, School of
Medicine, Omaha, Nebraska 68105

Purpose: To further elucidate cellular
abnormalities in cystic fibrosis, possibly
develop a test for the heterozygous state.

Subjects: Ninety cystic fibrosis
patients, ranging in age from 1 to 28 years,
miscellaneous hospital and clinic control
patients.

Methods: Lymphocytes are separated
from blood samples by glass bead column,
placed in tissue culture, stimulated with
phytohemagglutinin, radioactive methionine
added, and incorporation of radioactive
methyl from the methionine into RNA protein
and beta- glucuronidase is determined.
Samples are studied from both cystic
fibrosis and non-cystic fibrosis subjects,
also from heterozygous subjects.

Findings: Lowered beta-glucuronidase
level of phytohemagglutinin- stimulated
lymphocytes in cystic fibrosis.
Beta-glucuronidase appearing in two
fractions, one convertible to the other by
RNAase. First fraction being much more
susceptible to RNAase action in cystic
fibrosis than in controls.

MODE OF ADMINISTRATION OF PANCREATIC
SUPPLEMENT,
G.E. GIBBS, Univ. of Nebraska, School of
Medicine, Omaha, Nebraska 68105

Purpose: To determine conditions for
obtaining optimal benefit from pancreatic
enzyme preparations.
Subjects: Children with cystic
fibrosis.
Methods: Radioactive iodinated
triolein is given in 5 microcurie doses with
individual meals marked with carbon black.
The resulting stool is counted for
radioactivity to determine the percentage of
the triolein absorbed. Determination is
made of the effect of pancreatic lipase on a
particular meal as influenced by different
timing of the pancreatin dosage and
accompanying alkali.
Findings: No definite difference in
effect of pancreatin given before or after
meals.

MODEL OF CYSTIC FIBROSIS,
E.L. GREEN, Roscoe B. Jackson Mem. Lab., Bar
Harbor, Maine 04609

Cystic fibrosis is an inherited
recessive trait of human beings. It occurs
about once in 2,500 births and is fatal in
about half the afflicted children by about
20 years of age. Research on cystic
fibrosis is hampered by lack of an animal
model.
The purpose of this project is to
search for an animal model of cystic
fibrosis in the place most likely to yield

220

positive results; among the inbred strains
of mice, the mutant stocks of mice, and the
young sick mice, of all strains and stocks
at the Jackson Laboratory. The preliminary
results -- from mice with rectal prolapse,
electrolyte imbalance, and spontaneous
pneumonitis -- suggest that the search may
be rewarding.

The principal criteria of selection
are: previous history and inspection,
metabolic tests, and laboratory analysis.
Mice were deemed to merit further studies if
they had electrolyte abnormalities,
respiratory difficulties; sticky, fatty, or
loose feces; rectal prolapse or intestinal
obstruction. The metabolic test dealt with
differential ingestion of water and a saline
solution, weight gain, weight of food
consumed, and weight and characteristics of
feces produced. The laboratory analysis
includes activity of sweat chloride on the
skin of the foot pads, sodium and potassium
in hair, trypsin in feces, electrolytes and
amino acids in blood, urine, and fecal
material.

IMMUNOCHEMICAL INVESTIGATIONS INTO THE BASIC
BIOCHEMICAL LESION OF CYSTIC FIBROSIS,
S.P. HALBERT, Univ. of Miami, Natl.
Childrens Cardiac Hosp., Miami, Florida
33136

Cystic fibrosis is known to be a
congenital disease which is caused by
functional defects in many of the exocrine
glands. The essential metabolic disturbance
is not yet understood. The proposed work is
aimed at a comparative analysis of the
tissue constituents and body fluids of
patients with this disease, of
heterozygotes, and of normal controls in the
hopes of detecting significant differences

221

which might shed light on the basic
biochemical lesion. Since recent evidence
indicates that the ion activated ATPase
pumps of the erythrocytes from the patients
with this disease may also be defective,
emphasis will be placed on a comparative
immunochemical study of the proteins of
these cells which have been solubilized by a
variety of procedures. Attempts will be made
to identify the ATPase systems and other
enzymes in these immuno- diffusion reactions
by histochemical methods. It is hoped that
significant differences may be encountered,
as suggested by preliminary related work of
other investigators. Comparative studies
will be pursued on the presence of "tissue"
proteins detected in urine with antisera to
human submaxillary gland and pancreas.
Fragmentary evidence has been obtained which
suggests that cystic fibrosis patients may
have significantly different patterns of
these urinary proteins as compared to
normals.

PROTEOLYTIC ENZYMES IN CYSTIC FIBROSIS,
B.J. HAVERBACK, Univ. of Southern California,
School of Medicine, Los Angeles, California
90033

        The studies in this grant are divided
into four categories. 1) The separation of
alpha-2-macroglobulin into five components
with differing electrophoretic and enzyme
binding properties. Preparative acrylamide
gel electrophoresis separated
alpha-2-macroglobulin obtained from Bio- Gel
into 5 closely spaced species. Separation
was sufficiently adequate to show that those
species of alpha-2-macroglobulin which bound
trypsin and chymotrypsin were represented by
slower moving species and that the fastest
moving material had lost virtually all of

the ability to bind these enzymes. 2) Trypsin bindng alpha-2-macroglobulin in patients with acute pancreatitis. The serum trypsin binding activity was determined in 20 control subjects and 12 patients with acute pancreatitis and the values were 114 plus or minus 13 mcg of trypsin bound per ml of serum and 41 plus or minus 7 mcg per ml respectively (p greater than 0.01). The fact that the STBA of serum in acute pancreatitis is markedly reduced with the level of alpha-2-macroglobulin being unchanged, indicated that in this disease a substance, likely an enzyme, considerably in excess of the normal, is bound to the alpha-2-macroglobulin. 3) Kallikrein esterase associated with alpha-2- macroglobulin binding protein. Isolation and purification of alpha-2- macroglobulin revealed it to have esterolytic activity. Incubation with plasma substrate formed a kinin (bradykinin) which could be destroyed by chymotrypsin. 4) New trypsin inhibitory property of pancreatic tissue. Spontaneous and enterokinase activated trypsin activity was measured in isotonic saline homogenates of pancreatic tissue using BAPNA and RBB- Hide. Extracts from human pancreas, activated with enterokinase showed 9240 mcg of tryptic activity per gram of tissue when BAPNA was used, in comparison to 2220 when RBB-Hide was used. Activation of proteolytic enzymes by enterokinase in pancreatic extracts also activates an inhibitor different from Kunitz-Northrop's and Kazal's inhibitors.

PROGRAM PROJECT - RESEARCH IN CYSTIC FIBROSIS,
K. HIRSCHHORN, City University of New York, School of Medicine, New York, New York 10029

A primary objective of this

interdepartmental program project is to
elucidate basic defects in cystic fibrosis
through studies of the heterozygote. This
approach allows a search for primary defects
unhampered by secondary factors prevailing
in the homozygote. Our study has verified
the abnormal euglobulin found in the sera of
cystic fibrosis heterozygotes by Spock and
is attempting to provide a less tedious
bioassay for it. A concerted effort is
being made toward purifying and
characterizing both the abnormal substance
and the sodium transport inhibitory factor
described by Mangos. The effects of these
substances on membrane transport are being
studied, utilizing various in vitro and in
vivo systems. The relationship of
glycoprotein structure and composition to
membrane transport phenomena is being
studied. A second objective of this project
is to investigate developmental aspects of
lipid metabolism in crystic fibrosis through
studies of cell number and size and
parameters of fatty acid metabolism, in
order to determine any deviation from normal
development, and to enhance our
understanding of abnormal adipose tissue
development. A third objective to this
study will be to gain further insight into
the high gene frequency in cystic fibrosis
and to further quantitate its occurrence.
Simplification of heterozygote
identification is being attempted in order
to aid in genetic counseling, in
understanding the basic gene defect and in
developing human chromosome linkage maps.

CILIARY ACTION RELATED TO CYSTIC FIBROSIS,
T.L. JAHN, Univ. of California, School of
Letters, Los Angeles, California 90024

     The major objectives of this research

are: 1) To increase our knowledge of the physiology of cilia, especially those of the respiratory tract, in the hope of determining the role of cilia in the symptoms of cystic fibrosis, including the effects on cilia of the abnormal ionic ratios and the effects of certain organic factors in C/F and C/F heterozygote serum. 2) To screen protozoan ciliates for possible use as C/F heterozygote detectors.

STUDIES IN CYSTIC FIBROSIS,
H.G. KUNKEL, Rockefeller University,
Graduate School, New York, New York 10021

Efforts will be made to identify the cilia inhibiting factor from the cell line supernates. Purification of the factor is underway and comparisons will be made with the serum factor. Immunological methods will be utilized for further identification.

CELL CULTURES IN CYSTIC FIBROSIS AND OTHER DISEASES,
J.W. LITTLEFIELD, Harvard University,
Massachusetts General Hospital, Boston,
Massachusetts 02114

In this work it is hoped to increase the number of inherited disorders which can be diagnosed in fibroblast cultures so that these disorders can be studied in simple, well-controlled and homogeneous cell culture systems, and can be diagnosed prenatally with amniotic fluid cultures. In addition it is planned to study with the same purpose cultures of epithelial cells, which have recently become available here. Certain inborn errors or storage disorders may be

225

apparent only in epithelial cells. In
particular the cytoplasmic metachromatic
granules of patients with cystic fibrosis
may be more apparent in epithelial cell
cultures than in fibroblasts, since the main
manifestations of this disease involve
epithelial cells in vivo. Indeed a
distinction between the homozygous and
heterozygous states might be possible to
these cells. Finally epithelial cell
cultures will provide another tool for the
study of normal cell processes such as
senescence, differentiated function, and
cell-to-cell interactions.

STUDY OF EXOCRINE GLAND FUNCTION IN CYSTIC
FIBROSIS,
J.A. MANGOS, Univ. of Wisconsin, School of
Medicine, Madison, Wisconsin 53706

We have been studying: a) the
pathogenesis of the transport abnormality in
the exocrine glands of patients with cystic
fibrosis (C/F), and b) the function of
exocrine glands of rat, mouse and rabbit
utilizing enzymatic cell dispersion
techniques, micropuncture and microperfusion
studies and total gland functional studies.
We have demonstrated that the sweat from C/F
patients induced an abnormality of sodium
reabsorption when sweat glands from normal
subjects were perfused in vitro with sweat
from patients. In another study, it was
demonstrated that plasma or serum from C/F
homozygotes and heterozygotes inhibited the
uptake of 3-0-methyl-14C-D-glucose by rat
jejunal rings more than plasma or serum from
healthy controls. Finally, we have
investigated the secretion and transductal
fluxes of monovalent ions in the pancreas
and salivary glands of rat, mouse and
rabbit.

226

CYSTIC FIBROSIS AND PULMONARY DISEASE,
L.W. MATTHEWS, Case Western Reserve Univ.,
School of Medicine, Cleveland, Ohio 44106

The objectives of the two projects
included in this program project grant are
(1) to study the interrelationships between
cardiovascular and pulmonary function in
patients with congenital heart disease and
obstructive pulmonary disease, particularly
in the one month to five year age range, (2)
to develop and evaluate new methods for
studying pulmonary function in infants and
children, (3) to continue long term studies
of programs and measures for the provision
of prophylactic and therapeutic treatment
for cystic fibrosis, (4) to develop
clinical, bacteriologic, roentgenologic,
biochemical, pulmonary function test and
cardiologic methods for objectively studying
pediatric patients with chronic obstructive
pulmonary disease and (5) to utilize all of
these objective methods to assist in
developing and evaluating both new
therapeutic measures and comprehensive
prophylatic treatment programs. Individual
therapeutic measures which will be
specifically evaluated include inhalation
therapy, postural drainage, pulmonary
physical therapy, specific antibiotic
therapy and drugs which alter autonomic
control of pulmonary secretions, ventilation
and airway defense mechanisms.

CARRIER DETECTION AND SELECTION IN CYSTIC
FIBROSIS,
A.D. MERRITT, Indiana University, School of
Medicine, Indianapolis, Indiana 46202

Cystic fibrosis is the most common
autosomal recessive genetic disease leading

to high mortality and morbidity in man. The investigators have conducted research in families whose proband had cystic fibrosis. The following parameters are being investigated: (a) gene frequency estimate; (b) mutation rate; (c) number of loci; (d) penetrance; (e) differential fertility among carriers; (f) linkage analysis; (g) sweat chloride variability in cystic fibrosis families; (h) heterozygote detection (further evaluation of metachromatic granulation, biochemical evaluation of glycoprotein variability and their effect on bioassays involving ciliary inactivation). Family records have been carefully evaluated at the grandparent, uncle and aunt, and first cousin level. Data on 410 families is historically complete and has been rechecked at least once. Sweat chlorides on additional family members as well as extensive genotyping for erythrocyte antigens, enzymes, and genetically determined serum proteins for a total of 14 commonly polymorphic genetic markers are continually collected. Repeated, detailed family information verified within first degree relatives, their spouses and offspring, provide, we believe, the most accurate cystic fibrosis family data available.

In addition to the large scale population and linkage studies, several methods for heterozygote detection have been evaluated. Metachromasia in skin biopsies have proven reasonably successful but not cells derived from peripheral blood. The latter studies have not demonstrated genetically useful metachromatic granulation. Glycoprotein fractions from the serum and saliva are being tested in ciliary inactivation tests reported in oysters, mollusks and rabbit respiratory epithelium. Related studies of salivary glycoproteins suggest they may prove useful in heterozygote detection in either

biochemical or bioassay presently in
progress.

HORMONAL INFLUENCE ON CELL FUNCTION,
C.J. NABORS, Univ. of Utah, School of
Medicine, Salt Lake City, Utah 84112

We will study hormonal control of wound
healing and the cell cycle. Cell cycle
studies will also be done in cystic
fibrosis. Endometrial reproductive
endocrinology will also be studied.

BIOCHEMISTRY OF CYSTIC FIBROSIS STUDIED IN
VITRO,
H.C. PITOT, Univ. of Wisconsin, School of
Medicine, Madison, Wisconsin 53706

Work carried out under this grant
includes basic research of the
pathophysiology of inherited metabolic
disease, particularly cystic fibrosis (CF)
and hyperuricemia syndromes, utilizing
diploid human fibroblasts in culture.
Membranes from CF and control fibroblasts
will be examined for differential amino acid
incorporation and electrophoretic mobility.
Potential assay systems for the salivary CF
factor will be examined in an attempt to
isolate the secreted sodium inhibitory
material. Preparative starch gel
electrophoresis will be employed to see if
the salivary factor has a positive charge.
Cultured fibroblasts from patients with
hyperuricemia syndromes will be examined for
sites potentially responsible for
accelerated purine metabolism. The
overproduction of purines in man may result
from an attempt to overcome partial or near

complete metabolic blocks in the synthesis
of an important nuecleotide. Nutritional
studies will be used in fibroblasts with
inhibited de novo synthesis to study
potential blocks in the synthesis of adenine
or guanine nucleotides. Radioactive purine
precursors will be given to cultured
fibroblasts and the acid soluble nucleotides
extracted and analyzed by thin layer
chromatography. On the basis of these
studies specific enzyme reactions will be
evaluated in detail.

POLYSACCHARIDE METABOLISM IN CYSTIC FIBROSIS,
O.M. RENNERT, Univ. of Florida, School of
Medicine, Gainesville, Florida 32601

The objective of this project is to
detect possible differences in carbohydrate
and nucleic acid metabolism between
fibroblast cell cultures derived from
patients with cystic fibrosis (CF) and those
from control subjects. In the long term, we
hope to elucidate the underlying biochemical
defect of the disease.
Goals and Objectives of This Research:
1) To investigate the nature of the
metachromasia reported in CF fibroblasts.
2) To compare plasma membranes and
cell-surface glycoproteins from normal and
CF fibroblasts. 3) To test a number of
possible precursor compounds for use in
labeling complex carbohydrates in normal and
CF fibroblasts. 4) To investigate
methionine metabolism in relation to RNA
methylation in CF tissues.

RESEARCH ANIMAL DIAGNOSTIC LABORATORY,
J.H. RUST, Univ. of Chicago, School of
Medicine, Chicago, Illinois 60637

The diagnostic and research laboratory
has three functions and objectives (1) to
serve as a diagnostic center for diseases of
laboratory animals in the A.J. Carlson
Research Facility and other animal
facilities of the University of Chicago.
Capabilities of the diagnostic center
include autopsy, histopathology, hematology,
clinical chemistry, microbiology and
ultrastructural pathology. These are
utilized to diagnose disease outbreaks,
establish base lines of spontaneous disease
and to provide consultation on disease
control. (2) Serve similarly as a
diagnostic consultant and referral center
for biological and medical investigators in
the Chicago area. (3) Conduct such
investigations, studies and research as may
be necessary to improve the service of the
diagnostic center and enhance the art and
science of laboratory animal medicine.
Current research includes a study of animal
models for kidney and bladder carcinogenesis
research and models for cystic fibrosis.
Work also includes base line studies of
spontaneous disease in several species. The
diagnostic service is utilized in the
training of graduate students in comparative
pathology.

STUDIES IN CYSTIC FIBROSIS III,
H. SHWACHMAN, Harvard University, Childrens
Hospital Med. Ctr., Boston, Massachusetts
02115

To explore the basic defect in cystic
fibrosis through biochemical, biophysical,
and other methods.
To evaluate and improve present
therapeutic measures and to investigate new

methods with emphasis on pharmacologic agents.

To study all recognizable clinical complications particularly in young adults, infertility in males, biochemical alteration in cervical mucus, diabetes mellitus, cirrhosis of the liver as well as iatrogenic complications.

To detect the heterozygote by currently proposed techniques and to further explore tissue analysis for biochemical alterations in the parents and siblings of children with cystic fibrosis. To provide proper genetic counselling.

To improve and test procedures for detecting cystic fibrosis, simply, accurately and early.

To better acquaint practicing physicians and pediatricians with this disease, by arousing their suspicion to recognize cystic fibrosis early - prior to the development of irreversible pulmonary damage.

CELL ULTRASTRUCTURE AND FUNCTION, S.S. SPICER, Medical Univ. of So. Carolina, School of Medicine, Charleston, South Carolina 29401

One objective of the studies concerns the detection and in situ characterization of biochemically unfamiliar macro-molecules, such as mucosubstances and basic proteins in certain sites. Thus, current correlated biochemical and histochemical investigations are indicating the presence of heterogeneous organelles with a variety of hydrolytic enzymes in human placenta. Another objective involves localization of known biochemical components including enzymes and glycoproteins in cell surfaces. Insight into the function of particular cells or

cell structures will be sought from
correlated ultrastructural and cytochemical
observations. For example, current studies
are evaluating acid phosphatase in lipid
inclusions and secretory granules in the
secretory coil of the human sweat gland.
Finally the contemplated research will
undertake to apply new knowledge of cell
biology to investigation of pathogenesis of
lesions in certain diseases. Examples
include the demonstration of increased
junctional complex associated bodies in
sweat glands of patients with cystic
fibrosis, increased vacuolization in sweat
glands of patients with Hurler's disease and
altered mucosaccharides in chief cells of
patients with stress ulcer.

MORPHOCHEMICAL STUDIES, LIGHT & ELECTRON
MICROSCOPY,
S.S. SPICER, Medical Univ. of So. Carolina,
School of Medicine, Charleston, South
Carolina 29401

One objective of the studies concerns
the detection and in situ characterization
of biochemically unfamiliar macromolecules,
such as mucosubstances and basic proteins in
certain sites. Thus, current correlated
biochemical and histochemical investigations
are indicating the presence of heterogeneous
organelles with a variety of hydrolytic
enzymes in human placenta. Another
objective involves localization of known
biochemical components including enzymes and
glycoproteins in cell surfaces. Insight
into the function of particular cells or
cell structures will be sought from
correlated ultrastructural and cytochemical·
observations. For example, current studies
are evaluating acid phosphatase in lipid
inclusions and secretory granules in the

secretory coil of the human sweat gland.
Finally the contemplated research will
undertake to apply new knowledge of cell
biology to investigation of pathogenesis of
lesions in certain diseases. Examples
include the demonstration of increased
junctional complex associated bodies in
sweat glands of patients with cystic
fibrosis, increased vacuolization in sweat
glands of patients with cystic fibrosis,
increased vacuolization in sweat glands of
patients with Hurler's disease and altered
mucosaccharides in chief cells of patients
with stress ulcer.

IMMUNOCHEMICAL ASPECTS OF NORMAL AND
DISEASED LUNG,
R.C. TALAMO, Harvard University,
Massachusetts General Hospital, Boston,
Massachusetts 02114

Immunochemical and biochemical aspects
of the plasma kinin system and alpha
1-antitrypsin in man and animals will be
studied in general and as they relate to the
normal and diseased lung. The study of the
activation of the kinin system and the
inactivation of formed bradykinin will be
examined in vitro, in the isolated, perfused
dog lung and in patients with a variety of
disease states. Studies of cystic fibrosis,
carcinoid syndrome, dumping syndrome and
endotoxin shock will be emphasized.

The molecular basis for the different
known variants of the alpha 1-antitrypsin
will be studied. The significance of this
protein in the normal state, as well as in a
variety of pulmonary diseases will be
studied. Specifically, the role of this
protein in chronic inflammatory disease of
the cornea will be examined.

STUDY AND DIAGNOSIS OF HERITABLE METABOLIC
DISEASES BY USE OF CELLS CULTURED IN VITRO,
B.W. UHLENDORF, U.S. Dept. of Hlth. Ed. &
Wel., P.H.S. Natl. Insts. of Health,
Bethesda, Maryland 20014

In fibroblast cultures derived from
either human skin biopsies or human amniotic
fluid it has been possible to study
heritable metabolic diseases including
several types of homocystinuria, Hurler and
Hunter diseases, cystic fibrosis,
Niemann-Pick disease, and Fabry's disease.
Other heritable disorders are under study.

UPDATE AND COMPILE CYSTIC FIBROSIS
BIBLIOGRAPHY,
 UNKNOWN, Natl. Cystic Fib. Res. Found.,
Atlanta, Georgia 30326

Independently and not as an agent of
the Government, the Contractor shall update
the existing Cystic Fibrosis Bibliography,
initially compiled as a joint effort of the
National Institute of Arthritis and
Metabolic Diseases and the Contractor.
Specifically, the Contractor shall: 1.
Compile a comprehensive new Cystic Fibrosis
Bibliography by: a. Gleaning from world
medical literature all entries on the
subject of cystic fibrosis. b. Organizing,
indexing, and converting the citations for
printing by preparing copy-ready computer
programmed final tapes. 2. Distribute
approximately 10,000 copies of the
Bibliography, without charge, to individuals
known to be working in the field of cystic
fibrosis and related disorders, to medical
schools, departments of pediatrics and
genetics, medical libraries, nursing
schools, physical and inhalation therapy

235

departments, college and university basic
science departments, and other organizations
throughout the country.

FOR CYSTIC FIBROSIS RESEARCH EQUIPMENT,
 UNKNOWN, Long Island College Hospital,
Brooklyn, New York 11201

     No summary has been provided to the
Science Information Exchange.

SYMPOSIUM-CYSTIC FIBROSIS, GENETIC LUNG, AND
LIVER DISEASES,
W.W. WARING, Natl. Cystic Fib. Res. Found.,
Atlanta, Georgia 30326

     The purpose of the proposed conference
is to review, evaluate, and indicate
possible new directions for research in
cystic fibrosis and selected genetic
pulmonary, hepatic and pancreatic diseases.
Participation of basic scientists not
directly involved in investigations in these
disorders, together with researchers who
are, will permit objective evaluation of
completed research and should open new
constructive approaches to further study.
The conference will comprise two, and if
necessary three, daylong sessions: Day 1:
"Recent progress in C/F research". Day 2:
"Other selected genetic pulmonary, hepatic
and pancreatic diseases". Day 3: "Research
in the diagnosis and therapy of C/F".

236